12 Mo

MW00873522

12 Simple, Inexpensive Habits to Dramatically

Improve Your Quality of Life

By Jeremy Lesniak

I would like to extend a special thank you to Mr. Lester Nubla. Your many hours of perseverance and dedication to this project are what made it possible.

I also extend my gratitude to Mrs. Jenni Nather for doing … well … a lot.

Thank you, a million times over, my friends.

~Jeremy

Congratulations on taking the first step toward better health!

If you would like some encouragement and support on your journey, join us in our 12 Months to Health group on Facebook. We share additional tips and advice beyond what is covered in this book. It's also a great place to ask questions and share experiences with other folks who understand that better health happens one step at a time.

Scan below, or search for "12 Months to Health" in Facebook Groups.

Hope to see you there!

Dedication

I've thought long about how to dedicate this book. I could dedicate it to various martial arts instructors who helped me to see the value of consistent effort over long periods of time. I could dedicate it to various fitness instructors who helped me see paths forward when conventional "wisdom" told me there was no choice but pain or surgery.

But I won't.

Instead, I'll dedicate it to everyone.

I believe where we are, today, is the result of where we all were, yesterday. I'm the first to admit that the actions in this book aren't brand new, revolutionary, or earth shattering. Rather, it's a novel approach to seeing real results.

Let's stop looking for the magic pills, quick-schemes, and so forth. Let's recognize that real, sustainable results are the result of small changes made over time. If we're willing to do that, we can revolutionize not only our health, but any aspect of our lives.

Disclaimer

Everything we reference here is based on research. We did not conduct the research. We are not guaranteeing any results. Despite the safety of the recommendations in this book, it's important you approach every recommendation with caution, and an eye to safety. Standard suggestions of speaking with a doctor before implementing any of these apply. Always consult your physician before making any change, especially one that is dramatically different from what you do now.

NOTE: Any product purchase and/or usage put forward in these pages are merely suggestions. All manufacturer instructions regarding product usage should be followed. Speak with a medical professional before using any products.

Our intention in giving you the possible impact of the actions is simply to motivate you. Few people, if any, may argue against the actions we outline here. The goal in giving you the potential outcomes of taking these actions is to encourage you to stay consistent with them. By overwhelming you with all the great things that these actions can lead to, you'll be more likely to do them, and do them consistently.

And one personal note – you may receive some feedback from others saying these things don't work or won't work. Unless you're told an action is unsafe, trust the process.

Contents

Introduction 7

Forewords 8

How to Read This Book 13

Month 1 – Drink One Large Glass of Water First Thing in the Morning 15

Month 2 – Start the Day with Fat 49

Month 3 – The Beauty of Good Carbs 81

Month 4 – Get Outside 114

Month 5 – Grounding 146

Month 6 – Park on the Farthest Side of the Parking Lot 179

Month 7 – Keep Magnesium Spray in the Shower 212

Month 8 – Ashwagandha 246

Month 9 – Wear Blue Blockers (Light Timing) 278

Month 10 – Breathing 310

Month 11 – Meditate 342

Month 12 – Practice a Daily Affirmation 374

Closing 406

References 407

Introduction

This book is the result of a massive change in the way I view the world. While conventional media tells us that we can make substantial impact if we just buy a certain device, or take a pill, I strongly disagree. In the rare cases where those offerings actually do what they say, they also carry with them consequences that often out-weigh the change you wanted.

Instead, over the last 10 years of my life, I've implemented a variety of small changes to my lifestyle, from diet, to relationships, to fitness and health. These changes are rooted in the idea that small changes that are turned into unconscious habits lead to the best results.

You can't become a great runner by spending 24 hours, one time, running. Rather, it takes a commitment to running a bit every day, and so it goes for anything we want to do, hence this book.

It is my sincere hope that you will approach this book with an open mind, implement the 12 small changes I am recommending, and give them time to see the progress. Small changes are often difficult to see, until they've had time to take effect. It's entirely possible you notice nothing for the first few weeks, even months, but don't give up.

If you're willing to do what is asked of you for the full 12 months, I can promise you that you will see results and be in better health, and for some of you, even the best health you've ever known, all without devoting substantial time or money to the endeavor.

And once you've done this, you'll be able to do anything.

Forewords

As a licensed acupuncturist and practitioner of Chinese Medicine, every day I am seeking to treat the root of dysfunction in the individual before me. Upon investigation I often find that the reason this person is seeking care may be related to the habits or lack of habits they have created in their daily lives. Sometimes there are genetic tendencies to point to or accidents that have occurred. But more often than not, there are dietary habits, mental habits, or sedentary habits that this person may not even realize may be problematic. Or they recognize these tendencies are contributing factors but find it very challenging to change their ways.

Aside from using the tools of Chinese Medicine to help support change in the body, at times it seems equally important for me to point out the habits that may be supporting the dysfunction. The challenging part at times is how to offer this person the appropriate guidance that is practical for them in order to truly set them up for success. Mr. Lesniak's book so powerfully does this. He offers this simple and methodical guide for implementing key, health enhancing habits that are adopted gradually over a year. He shows the reader through short, daily bits of information as to why each habit is worth implementing. And these are simple habits to incorporate into one's daily life, whose benefits are based on the research he has gathered.

It is an incredible feeling to know you're taking care of your body through the choices you make and the actions you take each day. Mr. Lesniak has laid out a well-researched, simple, and gradual guide to real success in incorporating healthy habits into one's daily life. I look forward to sharing this with my patients as a partner in their journey toward better health.

Joshua Singer, Licensed Acupuncturist at River Street Wellness, Montpelier, Vermont

I was honored to be given a sneak-peek into Jeremy's book. It reminded me a bit of "My Utmost for His Highest" daily devotion, but for health purposes. We all struggle with making positive and permanent changes. I really like that Jeremy offers small reminders each day for why making a positive change is a good thing. I also like that Jeremy provides peer-reviewed resources for each statement to affirm his statements are rooted in scientific study.

Debi Stafford MSN, FNP-C

Habits, routines, and performance patterns. These are the things we do every day. As an occupational therapist, changing these things to optimize health and help us through our challenges is what I do.

It is easy to set goals and intend to do things better. Social media is full of one-liner platitudes of what we should and shouldn't be doing. It is easy to get overwhelmed by all the things we "should" and "should not" be doing. Setting just the right goal is hard to do, and starting with consistent, bite-sized, achievable goals is the way to achieve real change in your health.

Simply stating you need to do something is not enough. Jeremy breaks this down. He gives you clear instructions and various reasons why you might want to consider following them. He doesn't speak in absolutes and doesn't overwhelm. Each month has a clear theme, and each day reinforces that theme. I cannot speak to each chapter, as some of the suggestions fall outside of my area of expertise, but all of these suggestions are thoughtful and easy ... Bite-sized.

Irvin Eisenberg, Masters in Occupational Therapy, Structural Integrator and Owner of Resilience Occupational Therapy

1% at a time.

Sounds like a small and insignificant number, particularly when considering our own health goals. But I would challenge you. Consider that the plagues of chronic disease in the modern world occur in that fashion. 1% worse … every day … until you can't ignore it anymore. Type II diabetes does not occur overnight. Obesity does not occur overnight. Hypertension does not occur overnight. Heart disease does not occur overnight. These conditions are, generally speaking, the cumulative product of decades of us misusing and abusing our bodies. So then, is it reasonable for us to expect that our doctor can make it all go away in a 15-minute visit with a pill? And if not, what to do about it?

The health care that we all hope for is a non-event. How many times would you like to be in the Emergency Room next year? How many days would you like to be hospitalized in the next year? For essentially all of us, the answer to that question is zero. We want to grow old and not take medications, not have surgeries, only dying suddenly in our own beds in our sleep in our elder years. In that scenario, however, the health care system makes no money. How do we support hospitals that need to keep the lights on or nurses needing a paycheck when we don't require healthcare intervention?

The answers to that question could fill many more books, but for our purposes, it is important to understand that our health care system is largely response-based. We wait for something to break, be it your blood pressure or your pancreas or whatnot, and then we pay to fix it. And that payment is often quite steep. Time away from work, expensive medications, doctor visits, chronic pain, surgeries, hospitalizations. Perhaps the health care system will right itself, and perhaps not. Certainly not in the near future. But our healthcare system, as it is built, right now, is largely not designed to help you until AFTER chronic disease strikes. Even preventative health endorsed by your doctor is left to the small choices you make daily, by yourself, well outside of the walls of the clinic.

As such, I would applaud the reader of this book. In turning these pages, you are taking responsibility for your own health and the potential of positive change. You are making a choice not to go down, or continue to go down, the path of chronic disease. In considering the small things that you can do every day, you are taking a step towards positive change, towards a path that supports your life goals and dreams. Most things that most people want in their lives are more easily achieved and better enjoyed without the burden of chronic disease. By and large, this is only something you can do for yourself, and it is time all of us looked inward for solutions.

And so, dear reader ... press on.

Joshua T. White, MD, MBA, Chief Medical Officer, Gifford Medical Center

How to Read This Book

It's not often a book comes with instructions on how to read it. Seems a little strange, perhaps, but there is a reason this section is here.

This book isn't just something you sit down and read continuously, all the way through. It is actually a life-changing program. By reading and doing the things in this book, in the order presented and at the correct pace, you will build a solid foundation for dramatically improved health. If you read the whole thing at once and try to implement all of the changes at one time, it will become overwhelming and unsustainable.

Instead, this book is meant to take a year to complete. Each of the 12 lifestyle changes comes with an introduction to the healthy habit as well as 30 beneficial reasons to make the change, with one benefit provided for each day of the month. You implement one small change per month and spend the entire month understanding why it is so helpful by reading one benefit per day as you complete your new habit. This will reinforce your commitment to implementing that change by making it a daily habit. By doing so for an entire month, you are far more likely to maintain each lifestyle change as you transition into the following month, adding a new action to continue improving your health.

I will mention that as part of some of the lifestyle changes you are about to begin, you may wish to purchase certain products, like supplements for example. If you chose not to purchase the items right away, that is fine, but having the item for the month and using it daily is the intent of the program, and that is how the benefits will be presented in those chapters. We will give you a reminder to purchase these items so you have time to plan, and no, neither I nor anyone involved with this book will benefit directly from your purchases of these items. The benefit will be all yours!

It is my sincere hope that you will trust this process and accept that real, sustainable, impactful change does not happen overnight. There are no shortcuts to reversing the last years or even decades of habits you have built. We all want the secrets and the hacks to life that make us rich, beautiful, and successful, but they do not exist.

You've gone so far as to purchase this book. You might as well use it in the way that offers the best chance for success.

To your health!

Month 1 – Drink One Large Glass of Water First Thing in the Morning

We all know how important water is. We've been taught since we were kids that drinking enough water is important. Being dehydrated, even a little, has an impact. Severe or chronic dehydration can dramatically reduce health and even lead to illness.

The challenge is, we are often given conflicting information about how much water to drink, when to drink it, etc. You also have the people who are pushing you to drink a seemingly insurmountable volume of water. Who has the time or the space in their stomach to drink a gallon of water a day? It just seems too daunting to accomplish.

This is why you shouldn't do it.

When you try to do something that is too big, or too much, you're not going to succeed, which means you definitely won't keep going. Trying to make a gigantic change in your usual habits is not a sustainable way to create better ones. That's why, like the vast majority of the population, you're not going to drink enough water if you try to suddenly drink those high volumes daily.

Instead of thinking about how you're going to squeeze in a gallon of water for the day, focus on drinking a single, large glass of water first thing in the morning. Do it before your morning cup of coffee, or your meal, or anything else. In fact, you may find benefit in keeping a glass of water on your nightstand to drink first thing in the morning. No, sipping at it overnight and then drinking half a glass of water in the morning doesn't count. It certainly won't hurt, but for some of the benefits that we outline in the following pages, that water needs to be consumed after you are finished sleeping.

Think about it, you just spent however many hours asleep, not drinking, and basically getting dehydrated. The water you are about to drink will wake up your system, increase your metabolism, and help you set a pace for the day that improves everything.

When we look at the amount of water that various experts recommend for us to drink in a day, most people get pretty close. What experts are not really telling you is that the food and liquids that you consume have water in them, and that counts toward the goal. Drinking a single large glass of water first thing in the morning will push most of you over the edge for your daily water intake.

While we aren't going to be picky here about the kind of water you drink, please know that there are differences in water quality. If you are someone who doesn't drink much water now, don't even worry about the water you are drinking. Unless you're getting it out of an infected mud puddle, just about any water that you drink will be better than not drinking water.

Remember, you can survive for several weeks without food, but only a few days without water. Let's prioritize water, which is why it's the very first action in this book.[1; 2; 3; 4; 5]

Day 1 – Drinking Water May Reduce Your Calorie Intake

You might be reading the title of today's section and thinking, "Hey there's no way that drinking something as bland and unsatisfying as water is going to keep me from eating so much."

But, in fact, it can!

The place in your brain that tells you that you're hungry is actually the same place that tells you that you are thirsty. The signal to our body from our brain can be somewhat vague. That leads many people to eat when in fact they are thirsty, not hungry. By starting your day with a large glass of water as the first thing that you do, you give your body a better reserve of hydration so that you are less likely to receive this signal from your brain.

Of course, I am not suggesting that you skip breakfast, or that a water fast is a good idea. Restricting your intake of food below a minimal safe level in favor of drinking water is a silly, and even dangerous, idea.[6]

Day 2 – Drinking Water Could Improve Your Memory

There are a number of health benefits to drinking water that you likely already know about, but here is one you probably haven't considered: your memory. By drinking enough water, your brain is more likely to function properly, and that includes memory recall. The opposite can also be said; if you don't drink enough water, your memory could suffer.

If you're looking for incredible cognitive performance, or a healthy, real-world version of that pill from *Limitless*, just start your day with a big glass of water.[7]

Day 3 – Drinking Chilled Water May Increase Your Metabolism

Did you know that drinking water could improve your metabolism? There are two main ways this is possible. First, by drinking water first thing in the morning, you kickstart all of the biological processes in your body that require having enough water in the system to function optimally. Secondly, though it's not nearly as powerful as the original research made it out to be, drinking cooler or cold water does require a bit of energy expenditure in your body to warm it up. This is because your body can only utilize water that is at the proper temperature. If that water is too cold, it must get warmed up.

This doesn't mean that all of your water has to be cold. The key is simply to drink it. That first big glass of water in the morning is a sure move if you are looking to rev up the calorie burn throughout your day.[8]

Day 4 – Drinking Water Before a Meal May Help Reduce Weight

It probably makes sense, but how often do you drink water before you eat? If you drink a glass of water before your meal, including breakfast, you may not be as likely to overeat. This is because your body can only handle so much volume at once. When there is water in your stomach before you eat, your brain is going to get the signal that you have consumed enough sooner. By drinking that first glass of water right when you get up, it is likely that you will eat less than you would have otherwise when you do get around to eating breakfast – and you should eat breakfast.[9]

Day 5 – Drinking Water May Help Reduce/Eliminate Joint Pains

We live in a modern society that includes a lot of aches and pains, especially in our joints. The number of people taking over the counter and prescription medications to address these issues is staggering, but how many of those people are chronically dehydrated?

Joint function is heavily dependent on water. This includes all aspects of the joint, including cartilage. In fact, healthy cartilage is up to 80% water. If your body does not have enough water, cartilage, which is responsible for a lot of what goes on in our joints, is not going to function correctly. This may lead to pain. Ever wake up stiff and achy from a night in bed? Yet another great reason to start the day with a big glass of water.[10]

Day 6 – Drinking Water Could Help Prevent Dry Mouth

Does your mouth ever feel dry? This is a clear indication from your body that you need to be drinking more water. The physiological response of the body not producing enough saliva is what leads to dry mouth. Keep in mind, this usually isn't just from you skipping a little bit of water. This is a potential sign that you have missed out on quite a bit of water!

When you think about how your mouth feels most mornings after you wake up, you can likely relate to that dry mouth feeling. Yet another reason and reminder that we should start our day with a big glass of water.[11; 12]

Day 7 – Drinking Water Might Help Transport Oxygen Throughout Your Body

Did you know that the blood in our body is about half water? Given that blood transports oxygen, which is a rather fundamental component of being alive, being dehydrated is likely going to impact the efficiency of our blood and the transportation of oxygen. If you find yourself getting winded from simple tasks, or you are trying to increase athletic performance, having enough water is an easy way to address those goals. Start the day with a big, tall glass of water, and watch what happens.[13]

Day 8 – Drinking Water May Prevent Blood Clots in Deep Veins

Did you know that your blood, when properly hydrated, is less likely to clot? Whether we're talking about deep vein thrombosis or venous thromboembolism, blood clots aren't anything that any of us want to happen. While they aren't overly common, and while the occurrence is more complicated than simply not drinking enough water, proper hydration could be some great insurance.

Look at all these wonderful reasons that we're stacking up for why drinking just a single glass of water in the morning is beneficial![14; 15; 16]

Day 9 – Drinking Water Could Prevent Difficulty in Swallowing

Dysphagia, or difficulty swallowing, can affect anyone, though it's most common in older adults. Guess what may have an impact on keeping it in check? You guessed it, drinking more water. Get that first glass down first thing in the morning to set everything with your day on the right track.[17]

Day 10 – Drinking Water May Prevent Dry Skin

You've probably heard that your skin is the largest organ in your body. Healthy skin is about 64% water. When it is healthy, your skin does oodles for you, including maintaining temperature and preventing environmental toxins from entering the body. One of the ways that we know skin isn't healthy is if it is overly dry. What's the number one simple thing you can do to keep your skin hydrated and reduce dryness? You've probably already guessed, it's drinking water. That first glass of water in the morning is an easy way for you to keep your skin healthy and attractive.[18; 19]

Day 11 – Drinking Water Could Prevent Constipation

Nobody likes to talk about it, but your food has to go somewhere, and that includes the remnants of your food after your body is done processing it. Yes, we were talking about things that happen in the bathroom. Failure to drink enough water can have just as significant an impact on the tissues inside your body as on the outside. When your organs aren't hydrated, things don't move as easily. In other words, a dehydrated body may become a constipated body. While there are plenty of over-the-counter medicines that can help this, if you're not sure that you're getting enough water, you might consider this as a potential priority. Start the day with that first big glass of water and see what happens.[20]

Day 12 – Drinking Water Could Increase Performance in Exercise

Everybody knows that we sweat when we exercise. It's part of the body's approach to maintaining a healthy temperature. Of course, in order to sweat adequately, we need enough water in reserve in the body to produce that sweat. Did you know that if your body doesn't have enough hydration, it could compromise all of these systems and reduce athletic performance?

The time to drink adequate water is not in the middle of exercise, because that takes time to spread through the body. Rather, make sure you are hydrated before your bouts of exercise. Do you know the best way to start that process? You guessed it! A big glass of water first thing in the morning.[21]

Day 13 – Drinking Water Could Improve Mood

It seems like the older I get the more I learn about the various things that could impact our mood. I was surprised to learn that improper hydration is one of those things, and it carries a negative impact. Who knew? Well, now that we both do, it's yet another reason to drink plenty of water through the day.

Always start your day with that first big glass of water. Having a bad day? Try grabbing another glass of water and see if it helps.[22]

Day 14 – Drinking Water May Improve Decision Making

We keep accumulating these wonderful benefits of proper hydration! Keep in mind, it's not like your body is choosing one of them or a few of them – you get all of them!

Today, consider decision making. Studies have shown that dehydrated people are better able to improve their overall cognitive performance regarding judgment and decision making simply by drinking more water. Instead of waiting until you're dehydrated and allowing your work to suffer, start the day with a large glass of water and keep everything on track.[23]

Day 15 – Drinking Water Could Regulate Body Temperature

We've talked about sweat, blood, oxygen, and all sorts of other things regarding the blood in your body and how water might impact them all. By simply not having enough fluid in the body, you likely don't have enough blood. A lack of blood is going to restrict the body's ability to move heat around and properly maintain the optimal temperature.

Most of us were taught that the average human has a core temperature of 98.6F degrees. Some of the people who aren't operating at that temperature may be dehydrated. By not drinking enough water, your blood can become thicker, and your heart can work harder to process that thicker blood. Rather than expect so much of that all-important organ, just start your day with a big glass of water and give your body the support it needs.[24]

Day 16 – Drinking Water Could Prevent Drying of Eyes

We use our eyes so often, and for such basic things, that it's easy to forget they are an organ. As with any organ, not being properly hydrated is going to impact the proper function of your eyes. Dehydration can lead to dry eyes, which can produce symptoms ranging from discomfort to poor vision, or even worse. Rather than using eye drops exclusively, or frequently, consider drinking more water. I know that first glass in the morning has made a big difference in keeping my vision up as I have aged.[25]

Day 17 – Drinking Water Could Help Prevent Urinary Tract Infections (UTI)

While more common in women, anyone can get a urinary tract infection. This occurs when bacteria build up somewhere along the urinary tract. There have been some studies in nursing homes that found when residents were encouraged to drink more water, they suffered a lower rate of urinary tract infections. This makes sense, as it will increase the frequency with which we ... well, you get the idea. Don't forget that first glass of water right when you wake up![26]

Day 18 – Drinking Water Could Prevent Lightheadedness

Ever get lightheaded? I'm going to guess everyone has at some point. That lightheaded feeling may relate to blood pressure, and specifically decreased blood pressure. Remaining properly hydrated increases the volume of blood and thus it potentially raises blood pressure. Now, don't get nervous. This isn't going to push your blood pressure into unsafe territory. We're just talking about bringing things back where they should be, so make sure that first thing you do when you wake up is get that big glass of water.[27]

Day 19 – Drinking Water May Prevent Bad Breath

Everybody's breath smells bad when we wake up in the morning. Some people have it worse than others, but there is one simple thing that you can do to help reduce it. I'm going to guess you've already figured out what it is. Yes, stay hydrated! By making sure you are hydrated throughout the day, you will reduce the tendency towards bad breath. One of the reasons that our breath is a bit worse in the morning is that we aren't drinking any water while we're sleeping. Kick the day off right with a big glass of water and you'll most likely see your stinky breath get better … or rather, smell it get better.[28]

Day 20 – Drinking Water Could Prevent Kidney Stones

Have you ever had kidney stones? Fortunately, I haven't, but I have numerous friends who have. Each one has described them as being horribly painful. Some even require medical attention. Do you know one of the easiest ways to likely reduce the formation of kidney stones? Yes, the answer, just like with so many other things, is remaining hydrated. When you wake up tomorrow, think about how good you feel as you're drinking that first glass of water. Know that you're giving yourself so many benefits from that single, simple action.[29]

Day 21 – Drinking Water May Prevent Chapped Lips

Remember when we talked about water and the quality of your skin? For many of us, our lips are the first place that we show the signs of dehydration. If your body doesn't have enough moisture, it can't keep everything functioning the way it should, and that includes the skin of our lips. If you find yourself applying lip balm frequently, there's a chance that increasing your water intake could help. When you wake up tomorrow, think about that as you drink your first big glass of water.[30]

Day 22 – Drinking Water Could Help in Diarrhea Treatment

Unfortunately, we're taking another trip into the bathroom today. It's important for us to talk about it because today's benefit is about one of the leading causes of death globally: diarrhea. There are scores of illnesses that cause diarrhea, and with many of them, it's not so much the illness that becomes the cause of death. It's dehydration. When our body is unwell, we need significantly more water. While you are hopefully not ill as you read this, keep this in mind the next time you are sick. Most of us need more water than we get on a normal day, but if you are ill, you need even more than the normal amount. Get that big glass of water tomorrow morning and be thankful for all the things it does for you.[31]

Day 23 – Drinking Water Could Relieve Nasal Congestion

There's a reason that we're often taught to drink hot tea or hot soup while we are sick, and more specifically, when we are congested. It is because drinking warm liquid can help in decongesting the nasal cavities. Even though I'm not recommending that your first glass of water be warm, you could certainly follow up that first glass with tea throughout the day. If you are someone who suffers from congestion due to allergies or any other reason, increased hydration should be part of your strategy in addressing it.[32]

Day 24 – Drinking Water Could Prevent Tooth Decay

It's almost overwhelming how many things fall away in our bodies when we aren't properly hydrated. We talked previously about dry mouth and inadequate saliva leading to your mouth feeling off, as well as bad breath. Did you know that it can also lead to tooth decay? Having adequate saliva helps fight off the bacteria and conditions in the mouth that encourage tooth decay. In addition to all that other stuff like brushing your teeth, drinking enough water can help your mouth remain healthy. Be careful of smiling tomorrow morning while you drink that first glass of water, though. You'll probably lose half of it on your shirt.[33]

Day 25 – Drinking Water Could Prevent Eye Diseases

Remember when I said that proper hydration is necessary for the correct functioning of every organ in the body? Don't forget that eyes are organs! Dehydration can lead to a variety of eye conditions, including cataracts and retinal vascular disease. Eye health is important in modern society, and I've even noticed that when my eyes are dry, I can't quite see as well. What do I do to remedy that? I'm sure by now you know. I drink more water! Start the day with a big glass of water, and your eyes will thank you.[34]

Day 26 – Drinking Water Could Increase Semen Volume in Men

Here is another benefit that proves how beneficial it is to put these topics in a book. While it may not be considered proper to discuss publicly, adequate hydration has a strong impact on male sexual health.

Inadequate hydration can lead to reduced semen volume, as the primary component is water. It can also lead to a reduced libido and make erection more difficult to achieve or maintain. While there are certainly a variety of other factors that can impact these elements of male sexual health, if you are struggling with any of them, increasing your water intake may be a good place to start. Grab that big glass of water when you wake up, and you'll be good to go, in more ways than one.[35]

Day 27 – Drinking Water May Alleviate Depression

Your brain is an organ. As we've already established, every organ needs proper hydration to work correctly. This begs the question, what are the symptoms of a dehydrated brain? One of them is depression. I won't quote a statistic here, because the research is varied, but a great deal of people worldwide are chronically dehydrated. It's also no secret that a large portion of the population is depressed. Now, I am definitely not saying that all depressed people need to do is drink more water, but I can definitely vouch for my own experience. When I haven't had enough to drink, I don't feel at my best. The symptoms of depression that sometimes linger around the edges of my mind become more front and center. I've learned that by drinking more water, I can reduce and overcome these feelings. This is yet another great benefit of starting the day with a big glass of water.[36]

Day 28 – Drinking Water Could Be Used for Fasting

There are a variety of fasting protocols out there today, and intermittent fasting has become incredibly popular. While the idea of fasting is too complex for a book of this nature, it is something that I think everyone should research, and many people should try. However, unlike many others, I would never recommend fasting for weight loss. That's a recipe for building unhealthy eating habits.

Fasting has quite a number of benefits, and water becomes a significant component within fasting. We know that the body doesn't need food every day to survive, but even a short period of dehydration can have serious effects. While I have experimented with fasting in various forms, I have never done so without water, and I never would. In fact, some of the biological benefits to fasting require proper hydration for full effect.

If you fast, or plan to, or even if you don't have any desire to fast at all, you should still be drinking plenty of water. Water is the most important thing you can put into your body, so make sure you start the day by doing just that.[37]

Day 29 – Drinking Water Could Help Maintain the Ample Amount of Breast Milk

Improper hydration can have significant impact on not only the production volume of breast milk, but the composition of that milk. Dehydration, even small amounts, can lead to reduced lactose in breast milk. Lactose is the primary carbohydrate in breast milk and has been shown to improve a baby's ability to absorb certain essential minerals, including calcium. Obviously, not everyone reading this book will be breastfeeding a child, but when we consider that this is the root of our physical development, and water is critical in that process, it becomes obvious that water is paramount to everything we are. Don't take that for granted, but rather honor where we come from and start your day with a big old glass of water.[38]

Day 30 – Drinking Water Could Prevent Respiratory Failure

Do you know what our sinuses do? The main purpose of our sinuses is to produce mucus for the inside of our nose. Why? They do this to capture dust, environmental pollutants, and even microorganisms, so they can't enter our body. When we don't have enough water, our sinuses can't produce adequate mucus, and we may ingest more of that external gunk than we should be. A properly hydrated body produces an adequate amount of mucus and helps to keep us healthy. Gross to think about? Absolutely, but that doesn't change the fact that you should be drinking plenty of water. You might be getting sick of hearing me say this, but start your day with a single big glass of water.[39]

Key Takeaways

The hope, as you end this chapter, is that you are feeling overwhelmed at the sheer number of benefits that can come from just staying hydrated. Why are we focused on just one glass, first thing in the morning? It's because that is the easiest way to increase the amount of water you drink. Sure, I could suggest that you carry around a big water bottle, or schedule water breaks on your calendar, but everyone lives a different life, and many of us have complicated and busy, even stressful, days ahead of us. The goal here is to find a schedule that works for you, so that you are more likely to incorporate your new love of drinking water.

When the task at hand is simply to drink a big glass of water as the first thing you do when you wake up (within that first 15 minutes after waking for the most benefit), it is easier to make it a habit. Everyone has time for it, and everyone has water. It could help if you keep your drinking water near you, such as putting it close to your bed to make it easy to take that first drink when you wake. We could have spent a lot of time in this chapter talking about the different qualities of water, where to get the best water, and other details like that, but we didn't, because in all but extreme cases, any water is better than no water.

Our bodies, overall, are about 60% water. Our brain and heart are roughly 73% water. The lungs are 83% water, while skin is 64%. Muscles and kidneys are 79% water, and even bones are 31% water. When you think about everything we've lined up here, you might start thinking about drinking lots of water throughout the day, and I would absolutely applaud that action. If you have the time and the memory to do so, please, drink more water. It's hard to drink too much water, but for most people, drinking one big glass in the morning is going to make a pretty substantial difference, and that's the purpose of this book — to give you a running list of things to do that are easy, inexpensive, and overwhelmingly beneficial for your health.

As you move into the next chapter, don't stop drinking water! The whole point of this chapter was to build a routine around that first act of the day being your first big glass of water.

Hopefully, now that we are a month into this, you've established that habit and we don't have to talk about it anymore.

Month 2 – Start the Day with Fat

Most of the time, fats are perceived as the bad guys. Health buffs would usually tell you to stay away from fatty foods as much as possible. This is partially correct, but without the right knowledge on fats, you may misunderstand the significance of fats in the body.

Did you know that there are four types of fats? These are saturated, monounsaturated, trans, and polyunsaturated fats. These terms may be jargon to your ears but knowing the difference between these fats at least on a surface level would make you wiser in choosing foods in the supermarket.

If you are totally staying away from fats, we hope that this chapter will give you an idea of how important fat is in the body.

Day 31 – Healthy Fats at Breakfast Could Promote Better Metabolism

The advent of cereals in the late 1800s paved the way for a better choice of breakfast foods. Today, we usually put milk in our cereals which is high in fat. According to studies, the type of food you eat in the morning seems to affect your metabolism throughout the day. Therefore, if you eat fat-rich food at breakfast time, like cereals with milk, your body may have better utilization of fats for the rest of the day.

Milk does not contain just fat. It has plenty of other nutrients, such as calcium, magnesium, vitamin B12, and iodine. Unless you have a health concern, such as lactose intolerance, milk with your breakfast is a great way to get that serving of fat.

Even though your metabolism is programmed by the type of food you eat in the morning, you should still observe moderation. After all, we all have different activities throughout the day, and ideally, you should only eat what you can burn.[40]

Day 32 – Healthy Fats Could Reduce Blood Cholesterol

If cholesterol is a type of fat, how could fat intake lower blood cholesterol? Sounds ridiculous, doesn't it? Hear me out, though. Remember when I told you in the introduction that there are several types of fats? The healthiest type of fat is the monounsaturated fat that is found in olive oils and avocados, among many others.

Research shows that diets high in monounsaturated fats can reduce very-low-density lipoprotein (VLDL) cholesterol, which is a bad cholesterol.

Like I said, these healthy fats may indeed lower bad cholesterol. Neat, isn't it?[41]

Day 33 – Healthy Fats Might Be Beneficial for People with Diabetes

As you may know, diabetes can occur when your blood glucose is too high. If you are diabetic, it is very important to have self-control on food intake, as well as constantly monitoring your blood glucose levels.

The good news is that foods rich in monounsaturated fatty acids (MUFA) can improve control over the glucose levels and will not induce weight gain if the intake is in moderation. Also, studies show that MUFA-rich diets can reduce plasma triacylglycerol as much as 19% and VLDL-cholesterol (bad cholesterol) concentrations by 22%.

Feel free to use oils such as olive oil, sesame oil, and canola oil for your recipes. Avocados and nuts are also rich in monounsaturated fats, so you can have them as your snack or dessert.[42; 43]

Day 34 – Healthy Fats in Your Diet Could Promote Weight Loss

If you are trying to lose weight, you don't need to sacrifice all the fats. Did you know that monounsaturated fats can decrease body weight, body mass index, waist circumference, and body fat mass? Yes, it's true!

What you must avoid are the bad fats. These include pizzas, burgers, cakes, butter, margarine, fried foods, among many others. While these can still be eaten, these should not be part of your main diet, whether you are trying to lose weight or not.

Also, don't forget to exercise! Losing weight through proper diet is much more effective when accompanied by regular exercise to burn the calories.[44]

Day 35 – Healthy Fats Could Promote a Healthier Heart

Let's admit it, unhealthy foods are delicious, and we can't seem to live without them. In fact, according to a survey, pizza is the most sought-after food after steak, tacos, pasta, and burgers. We love these fatty foods, and many of us are not realizing their effects on our cardiovascular health. Not surprisingly, heart disease is the leading cause of death in the United States.

That's why it's high time to change our diets and make our health a priority. Don't worry, you don't need to give up all the fats. Results of a study show that a diet rich in unsaturated fat lowers blood pressure and triglyceride levels, which means a lower risk of having cardiovascular disease in the next 10 years.

Instead of pizzas and steaks, eat fatty fish (like salmon and mackerel), nuts, avocados, and seeds (like almonds and cashews). Healthy foods can be delicious, too! Sometimes we just have to be creative with our recipes.[45]

Day 36 – Healthy Fats in the Diet Could Decrease the Risk of Breast Cancer

Statistics show that about 1 out of 8 women in the US will develop invasive breast cancer during her lifetime. This is alarming because not only is this deadly, but the cost of treatments is expensive as well.

Numerous studies about breast cancer prevention are being done, and thanks to our scientists, they found out that increased intake of polyunsaturated and unsaturated fatty acids is associated with a decreased risk of breast cancer. On the other hand, a diet rich in starch is linked to an increased risk.

To women, I urge you to lower the intake of starchy foods such as pasta, white bread, and white rice. Eat more fruits, vegetables, and foods that are high in fiber, and work to include some healthy fats in your diet.[46]

Day 37 – Healthy Fats in Your Diet May Help Improve Insulin Sensitivity

You may not have diabetes, but you should be wary of developing it. If you think you have a sweet tooth and can't resist eating sweets, then my advice for you is to eat foods high in monounsaturated fats. However, for this to be effective, you should also decrease your intake of foods high in saturated fats, such as pastries, cakes, burgers, bacon, milk and white chocolate, butter, etc.

If you take this advice, your insulin sensitivity may eventually improve. That means your body could use the sugars in your blood (glucose) more effectively, thus lowering the risk of developing type 2 diabetes.[47]

Day 38 – Healthy Fat May Promote Good Mental Health

Who would have thought that fats can improve mental health? According to studies, diets high in monounsaturated fats increase the production and the release of the neurotransmitter acetylcholine, which is beneficial in memory and learning. Moreover, it has been found that people who have Alzheimer's Disease have a short supply of said neurotransmitter, so it's better to have enough acetylcholine especially at old age.[48]

Day 39 – Healthy Fats May Reduce Inflammation

Some studies suggest that diets high in monounsaturated and polyunsaturated fats could be anti-inflammatory. If you are suffering from inflammation, do not hesitate to eat avocados, nuts, and fatty fish, such as salmon and mackerel. If you want to maximize the benefits of these fats, you should consider consulting a physician, especially if your inflammation is severe.[49]

Day 40 – Healthy Fats Could Fight Depression and Anxiety

If you live in a place where a variety of oily fish is available, you should take advantage of it. Fatty fish, such as salmon, herring, and mackerel, are rich in omega-3, a type of fatty acid. Studies suggest that omega-3 is effective against depression, an illness that is suffered by at least 17 million adults in the US alone.

There are tons of delicious recipes for these types of fish. We're lucky the information is very accessible nowadays because of the Internet, and we can quickly search for these delicious recipes. I know many people are not fond of fish because, you know, they smell fishy, but you're missing out on a lot of health benefits if you don't eat them.[50; 51]

Day 41 – Healthy Fats May Promote Good Eye Health

Have you ever thought that fat is good for your eyes? It could be! Well, not all fats, but the one that is called omega-3. This type of fat is usually found in oily fish (like salmon, tuna, and mackerel), nuts and seeds (like chia seeds and walnuts), and plant oils (like soybean oil and canola oil). Yes, omega-3 can be found in many foods, but we seem to not eat them frequently, maybe due to availability or taste.

If these foods are easily available to you, I urge you to buy them instead of pizza, steak, or burgers. I'll throw some scientific terms here, but you can easily look them up to verify. There is what we call *docosahexaenoic acid* (DHA), which is a type of omega-3 fatty acid that is a major structural lipid of *retinal photoreceptor outer segment membranes* (photoreceptors are the cells that respond to light). DHA may alter the permeability, fluidity, thickness, and lipid phase properties of the photoreceptor membrane. It also affects the retinal cells involved in *phototransduction* (process of converting light into electrical signals).

In essence, foods high in omega-3 can be beneficial to our eyes in many ways, making sure that our eyes can see clearly and not be easily dazzled.

Also, studies have found that insufficient DHA can worsen the function of our retinas, so doctors sometimes give DHA supplementation to patients with visual problems.[52; 53]

Day 42 – Heathy Fats in the Diet May Be Beneficial to the Child During Pregnancy

If you are pregnant or trying to get pregnant, this information may be useful to you. In a clinical trial, pregnant women in their 18th week of pregnancy were made to take 10 mL of cod liver oil (which is rich in omega-3 fatty acid) or corn oil until three months after delivery. The results show that those who took cod liver oil had their children score higher on the Mental Processing Composite of the K-ABC at four years of age as compared with children whose mothers took corn oil.

Just imagine the effect of what pregnant women eat during their pregnancy to their children. While genes are a great factor to the qualities of the child, you should also consider that the foods you eat can affect your baby. That is why it is always a doctor's recommendation to eat healthy foods when you are pregnant. Remember that what you eat is also what the baby eats.[54; 55]

Day 43 – Healthy Fats May Reduce ADHD Symptoms in Children

At least six million children in the US are diagnosed with ADHD. If you have a child with ADHD, extra patience is needed as a parent to help them manage the symptoms. There is no cure for this disorder. There are several treatment options, like therapies and medications, but these could eat up your budget in the long run.

The good news is that studies have shown that fish oil supplementation may reduce ADHD symptoms. It doesn't always have to be an oral supplement. You can cook fatty fish, such as herring, tuna, mackerel, and sardines. You may consult your child's doctor about this to know the dosage if your option is fish oil supplement.

Do not give up on your child suffering from ADHD. I know it's a lot of work, but I also know that you're a loving parent who wants the best for your child.[56]

Day 44 – Healthy Fats Could Lower the Risk of Colon Cancer

Studies show that increased consumption of omega-3 polyunsaturated fatty acids may reduce the risk of colon cancer. Colorectal or colon cancer is one of the deadliest cancers because it does not usually display symptoms in the early stages, and most people do not undergo colonoscopy or other screening tests. That is why if you have the chance and the money to undergo these tests at least once a year, do it! Survival rate is a lot higher when treated in the early stages. Prevention is better than cure.[57]

Day 45 – Healthy Fats May Reduce Asthma in Children

It may sound absurd at first, but fats can help children with asthma. The long-chain n-3 polyunsaturated fatty acids (LCn3PUFAs) can reduce the risk of asthma development in childhood, according to studies. It is usually found in fish, but it is also in beef, lamb, and poultry. Fish is recommended to women and infants, but certain types of fish with high levels of contaminants, such as swordfish and tuna, should be avoided.[58]

Day 46 – Healthy Fats May Reduce Menstrual Pain

While most women experience slight discomfort during their period, there are some women who experience a great degree of pain, enough that it disrupts their activities. Sadly, it cannot be prevented, but there are some ways to lower the pain intensity, such as eating a balanced diet and doing regular exercise.

Did you know that foods that are high in omega-3 fatty acids are associated with milder menstrual symptoms? Thanks to scientific studies, you have more reason to include fatty fish in your diet if you want to relieve some of the menstrual pain.

You may take painkillers such as ibuprofen, but do not abuse it. Just stick to the recommended dosage, or else you may end up damaging your organs.[59]

Day 47 – Healthy Fats May Promote Better Sleep

Do you have children who have difficulty sleeping? Some studies suggest that diets high in *docosahexaenoic acid* (DHA), which is a type of omega-3 fatty acid, may improve sleep quality in children. Further studies are required to prove this, but as you may have read in the previous pages (and the succeeding ones), omega-3 has tons of benefits. You and your child will reap these benefits by starting your day with healthy fats.[60]

Day 48 – Healthy Fats May Help Treat Signs of Skin Aging

Who doesn't want to look young? Usually, we think to buy skin products to make our skin look younger, but maybe we haven't thought about foods that can do this as well. Studies show that diets high in monounsaturated fatty acids (MUFA) such as olive oil can prevent severe facial photoaging, which is premature aging of the skin due to frequent exposure to ultraviolet radiation, either from the sun or other sources.

If your job requires you go outside frequently, I strongly suggest that you incorporate MUFA-rich foods in your diet. Not only could you have glowing skin, but you will also experience the many other benefits of these healthy fats![61]

Day 49 – Healthy Fats May Help Control Blood Pressure

Did you know that almost half of the adult population in the US experiences high blood pressure? The American diet plays a huge role in this, as does a lack of regular exercise.

Having hypertension increases the risk of developing heart disease and stroke, which are both deadly. If you have hypertension, I urge you to manage it soon, even right away! Try incorporating foods high in monounsaturated fatty acids (MUFA) in your diet. Studies have shown that these fatty acids, which are found in vegetable sources such as olive oil and canola oil, can prevent adverse blood pressure levels in general populations.

I know fried chicken and pizza are more delicious, but as we grow old our bodies will not be able to process these types of foods the same way. Let us make it a habit to eat healthy foods and live a long life together.[62]

Day 50 – Healthy Fats May Help Individuals with Chronic Obstructive Pulmonary Disease

Chronic Obstructive Pulmonary Disease (COPD) is a type of lung disease that obstructs the airways causing long-term breathing problems. In biology class, you may have heard of *bronchioles* (tiny airways) and *alveoli* (air sacs). These can be damaged and result in COPD. Smoking and poor air quality are main causes of COPD.

There is no cure for COPD, but some treatments are available to delay its progression. Aside from medical treatments, studies show that eating foods high in saturated fatty acids can increase the lung function of patients with COPD.

It is no secret that smoking kills, but I understand the addiction. However, realizing how important and fragile your life is may help you stop smoking. Sit and contemplate. Ask for help from family and friends if you cannot do it alone. Let's all promote good health and long life![63]

Day 51 – Healthy Fats May Prevent Central (Abdominal) Fat Distribution

Did you know that having a big tummy can increase your risk of having a heart attack? You're more likely to have a major heart incident by as much as 79% if you have extra belly fat. Of course, not only your heart is in danger when you are fat, but all your other organs as well.

One way to reduce belly fat may be to have a diet that is high in monounsaturated fat while lowering your carb intake. A carb-rich diet can redistribute fat toward the abdomen, so stay away from pizza, pastries, white rice, fries, and other foods that are rich in carbs and bad fats.

I do not fat-shame people since there is a variety of reasons why a person is overweight. Some may suffer from depression resulting in an eating disorder, some are not well-educated by their parents that being fat isn't healthy, and some have genetic disorders which makes them more susceptible to gaining weight or even obesity, among other reasons. For those who are trying to lose weight, it's not too late, and it will take a lot of dedication if you want to have a healthier weight.[64]

Day 52 – Healthy Fats May Promote More Physical Activities

If you are a sporty person, or if your job is physically demanding, you may want to have more energy to keep going longer. While carbohydrates can give you the energy immediately upon ingesting, monounsaturated fats can increase daily physical activity and resting energy expenditure (REE).

REE is the rate of transforming food into energy (or metabolism) that is required to maintain the most important physiological functions in the body when you are at rest. In short, monounsaturated fats may allow your body to burn more calories even when you're not doing anything.[65]

Day 53 – Healthy Fats May Increase Semen Quality and Quantity

If you are planning to get pregnant, one of the things that you should look at is your diet and lifestyle. Both the male and the female are responsible in conceiving a child. While it is more common to conceive easily, some people can't conceive even after years of trying, and this is really frustrating, even heartbreaking, to aspiring parents.

For the men, sperm quality and quantity may be increased by diets that are high in omega-3 polyunsaturated fats, according to studies. However, you should also significantly decrease the intake of foods high in saturated fats, such as fatty meats, pastries, and butter, among many others.

Simply put, just be healthy altogether. Proper diet with regular exercise will bring so much benefit, not only physically, but also mentally.[66]

Day 54 – Healthy Fats May Prevent Psychotic Disorder Progression

Did you know that more than 50 million adults in the US suffer from a mental illness? This includes mood disorders, eating disorders, substance abuse disorders, anxiety disorders, personality disorders, trauma-related disorders, and psychotic disorders (like schizophrenia).

If you notice anything strange with your child, it would be best to have him or her checked by a doctor to get treatments as early as possible. While receiving these treatments, you can also include foods high in omega-3 polyunsaturated fats in the diet of your child. According to studies, these healthy fats can reduce the risk of progression to psychotic disorder in young people.[67]

Day 55 – Healthy Fats May Treat Schizophrenia

In the previous page, we've discussed that omega-3 polyunsaturated fats can reduce the risk of psychotic disorder development. If a patient already has a psychotic disorder, like schizophrenia, fats can still be effective. Studies have shown that diets high in *eicosapentaenoic acid* (a type of omega-3 fatty acid) are more effective in treating schizophrenia patients than diets high in *docosahexaenoic acid* (another type of omega-3 fatty acid). However, it is still best to consult a doctor for a professional opinion since this is already a serious mental illness, and we don't want to interfere with the treatment.[68]

Day 56 – Healthy Fats May Improve Patients with Bipolar Disorder

It is estimated that at least 2% of adults in the US suffer from bipolar disorder. While this type of mental disorder is manageable, it can be life-disrupting without the support of family and friends.

A study was made involving patients with bipolar disorder in which they were made to eat diets high in omega-3 fatty acids for four months. The results show that this diet improved the short-term course of the illness.

If you have bipolar disorder, it is best to consult a doctor to receive the best medications/treatments for you. In addition to those treatments, remember that food, not just medications, can help a person overcome a mental illness.[69]

Day 57 – Healthy Fats May Reduce the Effect of Psoriasis

You may not like the taste of fatty fish, or they may not be available to you. The good news is you have another option, which are fish oil capsules. Actual fish and fish oil capsules will each give the same benefits, so buy away! Another bit of good news is that fish oil supplementation could significantly reduce the itching, redness of the skin, and scaling in patients with stable chronic psoriasis.

I know that having psoriasis is hard and can destroy your self-esteem, but please don't give up. In addition to trying fish oil supplementation, there are lots of medications available to manage this skin disorder. See your doctor for more information.[70]

Day 58 – Healthy Fats May Reduce Liver Fat

Your liver has small amounts of fat, but excessive fat will result in *hepatic steatosis* (aka fatty liver). If not treated immediately, *hepatic steatosis* can lead to liver inflammation and then to liver failure.

According to a study, diets high in omega-3 polyunsaturated fats may decrease liver fat, though the optimal dose for it to be effective is currently unknown. Consult a physician immediately to undergo treatments if you have a fatty liver.[71]

Day 59 – Healthy Fats in the Diet May Delay Brain Function Decline in Elderly Men

As we grow old, it is inevitable that our entire body becomes weaker, including our brain. Thanks to scientific research, moderate intake of *eicosapentaenoic acid* (EPA) and *docosahexaenoic acid* (DHA) from fish and other foods may postpone cognitive decline in elderly men.

Even if you aren't an elderly man, I'm hopeful that you are enjoying the numerous potential benefits of healthy fats in your diet.[72]

Day 60 – Healthy Fats May Decrease Fracture Risk

Our bones can become fragile depending on what we eat, especially as we become old. Usually, we think of calcium to strengthen our bones, but did you know that fats can also be beneficial to the bones? Studies show that diets high in monounsaturated and polyunsaturated fats may decrease total fracture risk as opposed to diets high in saturated fats, which may significantly increase hip fracture risk.

Yes, it is still important to have enough calcium and magnesium in the body to strengthen our bones. Now you know that healthy fats can also play an important role in our bone health.[73]

Key Takeaways

Remember that not all fats are bad, the same with carbohydrates which is discussed in another chapter. The ones that we should avoid, or limit, are the foods high in trans-fat and saturated fat. On the other hand, the ones that we should eat are the foods high in unsaturated fat (monounsaturated and polyunsaturated).

I know that many of us fry foods because 1) frying does not take much preparation and time, and 2), frankly, they are tasty. When buying cooking oils, buy the ones that are rich in monounsaturated fats, such as canola oil and olive oil. Olive oils are usually used in salads and not in deep frying because they are a lot more expensive than canola oil. They may be more expensive, but they are a lot healthier!

Also, I urge you to eat more fish than red meat. Oily fish such as salmon and mackerel are high in omega-3 fatty acids, which brings many benefits in the body as we have discussed in this chapter. An **important** reminder: pregnant women should avoid fish that are high in contaminants such as tuna, which can be high in mercury. Pregnant women should always consult their doctors first about their diets as some pregnancies are high-risk.

The benefits of unsaturated fats have long been established, but it seems that when people hear the word "fat", they immediately think that it is bad. No, our body *needs* fat. We just have to control our intake and choose which fats to eat.

Month 3 – The Beauty of Good Carbs

People have been consuming carbohydrates for thousands of years. Corn, rice, and wheat are examples of foods that are rich in carbohydrates. The cereals we eat in the morning, the bread in the sandwiches, burgers, and pizzas, the different kinds of pasta – these are all rich in carbohydrates.

Carbs are the body's main source of energy. Did you know that if you don't consume carbs, your body would utilize fat and protein instead? Carbs are the ones that digest very quickly, however, to give you that boost of energy, while fat digests the slowest.

You may have heard of diets that discourage carb intake. One example is the ketogenic diet (or keto diet). This particular type of diet focuses on eating fats instead, but does this mean that carbs are bad? In this chapter, we'll discuss the health benefits of carbs that people may not know.

Day 61 – Good Carbs May Help You Lose More Weight

Scientists performed an experiment involving 78 police officers wherein carbohydrates were eaten mostly at dinner over the course of six months. The results show that there was greater weight loss, waistline reduction, and body fat mass reductions. This study is controlled, of course, and the carb intake was in moderation.

Did you notice something? We usually eat carbs in the morning. Cereals and bread are rich in carbs! In this study, carbs were eaten mostly at dinnertime. You may try this experiment yourself (eating carbs with dinner rather than for breakfast), but do not overeat! Also, you must note that in this experiment, the participants were all police officers who are usually physically active, so keep in mind that along with proper diet, a proper exercise routine is needed to achieve optimum results.[74]

Day 62 – Good Carbs Can Help Provide Energy

If you are extremely hungry, carbs are the best (and probably cheapest) way to have that immediate boost of energy since they digest quickly. After just several minutes, you will feel the energy rushing through your veins and you will be able to move again.

If you are going on a long drive perhaps, prepare some sandwiches, or any easy-to-eat carbs. Never drive hungry because hunger can cause dizziness, and you don't want to be dizzy while driving![75]

Day 63 – Good Carbs Can Provide Stored Energy for Later Use

Did you know that your body can store energy for later use?
When you eat carbs, they are broken down into glucose. If you
have excess glucose, your body can store it for later use as
glycogen, but does this mean that we should eat a lot of carbs?
Nope. As with all other foods, we should eat carbs in
moderation. If your body's glycogen storage becomes full, all the
excess glucose will be stored as fat. However, you should not
worry if you eat excess carbs *sometimes*, because fat is still essential
to the human body. (Review the chapter on fats!)[76]

Day 64 – Good Carbs May Prevent Loss of Muscle Mass

When your body does not have something to digest due to prolonged starvation, it will resort to "eating up" the muscle cells to provide enough energy for the brain. Since carbs are easily digested, it can immediately help the body to use the newly ingested carbs and not the muscle cells.

If you are fasting (not intermittently), you may expect loss of muscle mass. Also, be mindful of your body's limitations to avoid any life-threatening situations. Eat right away if you think you are going to collapse. If you are living alone, I would suggest intermittent fasting rather than eating nothing for several days.[77; 78]

Day 65 – Good Carbs in the Diet May Prevent Constipation

Constipation is not typically life-threatening, but at the same time, it should not be ignored. If you want to get rid of constipation, you can eat complex carbohydrates such as soluble fibers, which are found in oats, carrots, and citrus fruits, among many others. Complex carbs are backed up by research to aid in treating and preventing constipation. Make a habit of eating a healthy diet which incorporates the right carbs, and you will not be constipated![79]

Day 66 – Good Carbs May Prevent Diverticular Disease, or Diverticulosis

Diverticulosis is a disease wherein the colon has multiple pouches, or *diverticula*. This disease is observed to be more common in Western populations, most probably due to low fiber intake. It is not usually a very serious disease, but it could lead to complications if not treated or managed immediately.

Scientific studies show that high intake of insoluble fiber (a type of complex carbohydrates) can lower the risk of developing the disease by as much as 37%. Foods rich in insoluble fiber include whole grains, cauliflower, green peas, and dark leafy vegetables, among many others.

From now on, try to include insoluble fibers in your diet. If we just eat tasty foods which are usually unhealthy, we will find ourselves sick sooner or later.[80]

Day 67 – Good Carbs May Reduce the Risk of Type 2 Diabetes

Studies show that eating high amounts of fiber, especially cereal fiber, can significantly lower the risk of developing type 2 diabetes. If you already have this disease, it is much more advised for you to eat high amounts of fiber. Fiber can slow sugar absorption, making it easier to control your blood sugar levels.

If you are fond of cereals, good for you! Continue eating healthy cereals because it can bring many benefits to the body.[81]

Day 68 – Good Carbs Can Lower Blood Sugar (Glucose)

We've learned in the previous page that eating fiber can reduce the risk of developing type 2 diabetes. Carbs are broken down into glucose (the main type of sugar in blood), so how can fiber (a type of carbohydrate) lower the glucose in the body? In other words, how can sugar lower blood sugar? Let me explain a little bit more about fiber's effects on blood sugar levels.

Dietary fibers, such as oat and barley, are rich in what we call resistant starch. This type of starch is resistant to digestion and beneficial to the gut bacteria, unlike the rapidly digested starch which is easily converted into glucose. Oat and barley foods that contain at least 4 g of β-glucan (beta-glucan) and 30-80 grams of available carbohydrates can significantly reduce the blood sugar after a meal. Barley has the highest beta-glucan content while oat ranks second.

Apologies for the jargon. The point here is that dietary fiber can bring you tons of health benefits, so you should consider including it in your diet.[82]

Day 69 – Good Carbs Could Help Provide Satiety or Fullness

One of the main reasons why we may become overweight is because we eat frequently, and most of the time the foods that we eat are not healthy. One effective and healthy way to solve that is by eating foods rich in dietary fiber. Since dietary fibers are slowly digested – which delays gastric emptying, or the time it takes for the stomach to be empty – it can make you feel full longer and eliminate the cravings.

Instead of white bread, buy wheat bread. Instead of white rice, buy brown, red, or black rice. I understand that the healthier options are usually more expensive, and I won't force you to spend beyond your means. If you have the budget, try to buy the healthier products and experience their wonderful effects in your body.[83; 84]

Day 70 – Good Carbs Can Promote Healthy Bowel Movements

Dietary fiber has two main components: soluble and insoluble fiber. It's quite self-explanatory based on their names. Soluble fiber dissolves in water while insoluble does not. They are both healthy, but since they differ in characteristics, their effects in our gut are different, too. Both are effective in treating constipation, but soluble fiber can improve stool consistency through its viscosity and water retention throughout the process of digestion.

Examples of foods high in soluble fibers are black beans, lima beans, brussels sprouts, avocados, sweet potatoes, broccoli, turnips, pears, apples, carrots, oats, and barley.[85; 86]

Day 71 – Good Carbs Can Provide Energy to the Brain

Did you know that, among all our organs, our brain consumes most of our body's energy? It's true! Even though it's only 2% of our bodyweight, it consumes about 20% of our energy! That's how demanding our brains are.

To be more accurate, the brain consumes about 5.6 mg glucose per 100 gram of brain tissue per minute. Our brain needs glucose to function properly, and the carbs that we eat are 100% converted to glucose. We can also get glucose from protein and fat, but only small amounts of them can be converted to glucose.

According to Dr. Ashish Shrivastav, a senior consultant neurosurgeon at Apollo Hospitals, "Carbohydrates are the only nutrients which can match this rate of energy requirement. However, the brain prefers to get its carbohydrates from carbohydrate rich whole foods rather than simple sugars."[87; 88]

Day 72 – Good Carbs Can Lower the Risk of Colon Cancer

Dietary fiber, which is one of the complex carbohydrates, is effective in reducing the risk of developing colorectal (colon) adenoma and cancer. This was proven by a large study involving thousands of individuals who were made to consume high amounts of dietary fiber, particularly from cereals and fruit.

Colon cancer is one of the deadliest cancers in the world, and as much as possible, we want to stay away from it. From now on, let us make it a habit to eat fiber-rich foods and live a healthy life, not only for us, but also for our loved ones.[89]

Day 73 – Good Carbs Could Lower the Risk of Breast Cancer

Breast cancer is common in the US, and one of the observed reasons is the lifestyle of women, including their fiber intake. Eating fiber is associated with reduced risk of the disease.

In some European regions and the US, the intake of dietary fiber is only about 22 grams a day, which is far below the recommended intake. Total dietary fiber intake should be at least 25 to 30 grams a day from food, not from supplements.

One of the functions of dietary fiber is absorbing the ions and organic compounds as well as free estrogen formed by human intestinal microbial enzymes, which may reduce the risk of breast cancer. Also, the fiber can reduce the level of female mammary hormones in the blood, which reduces the occurrence of breast carcinoma.

Let us take care of our health and promote a healthy lifestyle to the community. Always eating unhealthy foods is not worth it if we die early.[90]

Day 74 – Good Carbs Can Lower the Risk of Stroke

According to statistics, someone dies from stroke in the US every four minutes. That's how common stroke is, even though it is preventable and curable.

While there are many causes of stroke, the most common cause is an unhealthy lifestyle. Being physically inactive, eating lots of fats, and binge drinking are just some of the risk factors of developing a stroke.

If you don't want to experience stroke, change your diet into a healthy diet. Eating foods rich in fiber can reduce the risk of developing various diseases that could cause stroke, such as hypertension and diabetes.[21]

Day 75 – Good Carbs in Your Diet Might Lower Cholesterol Levels

Cholesterol is required by the body, but too much of it is bad for the heart. If you eat lots of beef, lamb, pork, chicken skin, and other foods that are high in saturated fat, you could see an increase in your cholesterol levels.

Studies have shown that increasing the intake of foods high in soluble fibers can help lower bad cholesterol or LDL (low-density lipoprotein) cholesterol levels. If you are currently suffering from high cholesterol, the first thing you should do is to avoid foods that can aggravate it and eat the foods that can lower it. You should also see a doctor to develop a plan for your healthcare. [92; 93]

Day 76 – Good Carbs in the Diet May Prevent Heart Problems

There are many reasons why a person develops cardiovascular disease (CVD). Some of these are high blood pressure, high cholesterol, smoking, diabetes, not being physically active, and obesity.

Studies are still ongoing regarding the effect of dietary fiber in the disease. However, several observational findings report lower incidence of coronary heart disease in persons who report consuming diets high in fiber. This is not surprising because dietary fiber can help prevent the causes of CVD, such as high cholesterol.

Sadly, CVD is very common. In the US, statistics show that a person dies of CVD every 36 seconds. It's about time we change for the better and live a long and healthy life.[94; 95]

Day 77 – Good Carbs Can Be Beneficial Against Systemic Inflammation

People suffering from systemic inflammation are most likely to develop inflammation-associated diseases, such as cardiovascular disease and diabetes. This condition could worsen by smoking, unhealthy diet, and hypertension, among others.

A study shows that whole-grain foods have beneficial effects against systemic inflammation in obese children. If you have an obese child, help him/her change his/her diet. Also, carefully explain the health complications that could arise from being obese. As parents, we are responsible for our children's health. Let us monitor what they eat, but we must also be role models to them.[96]

Day 78 – Good Carbs Can Promote Longer Life

According to statistics, heart disease is the leading cause of death in the US, followed by cancer and accidents. While cardiovascular disease can be inherited, its risk of occurring can be drastically lowered by maintaining a healthy weight and eating a healthy diet.

In fact, two large prospective cohort studies show that higher whole grain consumption is associated with lower total and cardiovascular disease mortality in the US.

Whole grains are affordable, and a lot more affordable compared to steaks and cakes. Let us not allow this disease to take away our lives too soon. If we love our families, we should do our best to stay healthy so we can be there for them as long as possible.[97]

Day 79 – Good Carbs May Help Redistribute Fat

Science shows that having excessive belly fat is not healthy at all. In fact, having huge bellies increases our risk of having cardiovascular disease and Alzheimer's disease, among many others. This is not about body shaming, but about your health.

Americans love alcohol and fatty foods. Combine these two, you will make it difficult for your liver to do its job since it will become fatty as well. Turn away from these unhealthy foods as much as possible and replace them with whole grains. These may help redistribute body fat instead of going all to the belly.[98]

Day 80 – Good Carbs in the Diet Can Be a Great Source of B Vitamins

B vitamins have tons of contributions in the body, such as in the release of energy from carbohydrates, metabolism, and beta oxidation. Whole grains are rich in them. True, these affordable grains are not necessarily as tasty as your favorite foods, but it could keep you away from serious diseases.

Nowadays, food delivery is very much widespread, especially in the cities, and almost any type of food is within our reach. Sadly, most of these foods are unhealthy, and the healthy ones are often unbelievably expensive. Try going to the supermarket, buying the healthy ingredients, and cooking the dishes at home. It can be more budget-friendly, but it can also help you eat better.[99]

Day 81 – Good Carbs May Reduce the Risk of Asthma

There are about 25 million Americans who have asthma in the US. Having this disease requires you to be very careful to prevent flare-ups, and you will need immediate treatment or relief as it can be life-threatening.

Studies show that eating whole grains early in life can reduce the risk of asthma and allergic rhinitis. For parents who have young children, take note of this. Encourage your child to eat whole grains. You can mix them with fruits and milk to add flavors. Most importantly, do not let them eat processed foods frequently. Hot dogs, bacon, nuggets – they are all unhealthy. The air that we breathe is often heavily polluted, so we should be more careful about what we eat.[100]

Day 82 – Good Carbs May Promote Gum Health

If you have persistent bad breath, chances are you have gum disease. You should consult your dentist right away to have it treated.

If you have never had gum disease, or you had it before and have since been treated, I have good news for you. A large study participated in by nearly 35,000 men showed that those who consumed the highest amount of whole grain were less likely to develop gum disease by 23%.

Of course, keeping your teeth clean is still the most important thing to do to prevent any gum diseases. Obesity is another risk factor. You can help reduce your risk of obesity if your diet consists of high-fiber foods and if you have good eating habits.[101; 102]

Day 83 – Good Carbs in the Diet May Promote Better Magnesium Absorption

Magnesium is very essential to the body. It helps with calcium absorption, and hence magnesium helps our bones become stronger and prevents loss of bone mass. Therefore, we need to make sure that magnesium is properly absorbed by the body.

The good news is that magnesium absorption is found to be improved by consuming dietary fiber-rich foods, particular those with high potential fermentability, such as bread and cereals. Eating foods high in fiber will help your body to build stronger bones, which becomes more important as we age.[103]

(We will talk more about magnesium later in this book!)

Day 84 –Good Carbs May Protect Against Bone Loss at the Hip in Older Men

Older people are prone to fractures due to bone loss, so there is a great need for them to have a healthier diet and regular exercise. The good news is that according to a study, dietary fiber and fiber from fruits may protect against bone loss at the hip in older men, but not in older women. Even though this was not found to be the case for older women, fiber still brings a lot of other benefits to the body, so ladies should still be mindful of their fiber!

Today's benefit is related to the previous benefit we discussed. Since fiber-rich foods help with magnesium absorption, and magnesium helps with calcium absorption, this type of diet can be more helpful for older adults to prevent bone loss.[104]

Day 85 – Good Carbs in the Diet Can Promote a Healthy Liver

Our liver has many important functions such as metabolism of carbohydrates, protein, and fats; storing glycogen; detoxifying the blood; and many more. We really must take care of our liver, or else we'll end up having many health problems.

According to a study, oatmeal and oats that contain beta-glucans reduce the amount of fat in the liver in mice. This may have the same effect in humans.

If you really want to keep your liver healthy, do not overeat. Excess calories will build up fat in the liver and may progress to a liver disease if not managed or treated early.[105]

Day 86 – Good Carbs May Help Improve Sperm and Testosterone Production

If you are trying to get pregnant, eat more fiber! Studies show that fiber-rich carbs can help sperm and testosterone production. However, if you have been trying for some time and still can't conceive, it's better to have yourselves checked by a doctor to get a proper and professional diagnosis.[106]

Day 87 – Good Carbs Can Lower the Risk of Infertility in Women

In one study, one of the results shows that an increase in cereal fiber intake of 10 g per day, while holding caloric intake constant, was associated with a 44% lower risk of ovulatory infertility among women older than 32 years. This is great news for women over 32 who are trying to conceive. Taking fertility vitamins, such as folic acid and omega-3 are very much recommended, but do not forget to have a healthy diet altogether.[107]

Day 88 – Good Carbs May Increase Bone Mineral Density

We are more familiar with milk supporting stronger bones. However, it's not the only food that we should eat if we want to make our bones healthy.

Studies have shown that diets rich in prebiotic fiber, such as fruit pectin, can improve calcium absorption and inhibit osteoclast (cells that degrade the bone) bone resorption, while maintaining osteoblast (cells that form new bone) bone formation activity. In other words, eating carbs from fruits is very beneficial to bone health. Apples are one of the fruits that offer pectin that has many health benefits, such as lowering cholesterol.[108]

Day 89 – Good Carbs Could Reduce the Risk of Having Crohn's Disease

Crohn's disease is a type of inflammatory bowel disease (IBD) that may affect any part of the gastrointestinal (GI) tract, which is from mouth to anus. This can lead to having severe diarrhea, fatigue, and abdominal pain, among other issues. Studies show that increased fruit fiber intake can reduce the risk of developing Crohn's disease.

Also discovered, those who regularly smoke are twice as likely to develop this disease. If you're thinking that smoking only destroys the lungs, you are gravely mistaken. I know smoking is addictive, but please be informed of the health implications not only to you but also to the people who inhale your smoke.[109]

Day 90 – Good Carbs Can Promote Psychological Well-Being

The microbiota in our bodies consists of bacteria, archaea, protists, fungi, and viruses. There are trillions of them, and they are found to affect our immune system, brain, and behavior.

Fiber-rich, healthy diets can positively impact our psychological well-being by improving the microbiota health. On the other hand, low fiber intake can increase the risk of impaired microbiota, which could cause a variety of health problems.[110]

Key Takeaways

There are types of carbohydrates that we should limit, such as cakes, pastries, and pizza. These are all delicious, right? However, these foods are easily converted into sugar, so too much of these can lead to diseases, such as obesity and diabetes. If you already have diabetes, it is advised to lower your carb intake by at least 50%, since carbs can spike your blood sugar.

On the other hand, the healthier types of carbs are the ones that are rich in fiber. These are found in whole fruits, vegetables, whole grains, nuts, and many more.

We must understand that carbs are the number one energy source of our body. They are easily digested, so eating these can give you energy quickly, as opposed to proteins and fats that digest slower.

I hope that this chapter gave you enough information to understand how carbohydrates are crucial to one's health. Always remember that the key to a healthy life is good diet and regular exercise. Also, stay away from vices that can easily harm your body permanently.

Hello!

When we reach Month 5, we will be discussing the benefits of grounding. There is a product called a grounding mat that will be mentioned. Feel free to research/shop and consider purchasing a grounding mat so you have yours in time for Month 5.

I will say that it is perfectly okay not to buy this item. Grounding can still be done without this product, so you will not miss out on the benefits if you do not make this purchase.

Now, go ahead and get into Month 4!

Month 4 – Get Outside

"There's no place like home."

I believe that most of us are still more comfortable staying at home rather than going somewhere else. Even if we stay at a luxurious hotel, there is still a feeling of comfort and belongingness in our own homes. Sometimes, we love staying at home so much that we don't want to go outside anymore.

If we stay at home most of the time, it also means that we are less exposed to sunlight. You might say, "What's wrong with that?" While it's true that humans can survive without sunlight for years, the health effects could be drastic. The last thing we want is to develop serious illnesses just because we didn't take the time to go outside.

If you have your own backyard, rooftop, or balcony where you can enjoy the sunlight, that is great, and I hope you are taking advantage of it! However, there are still millions of people, especially those who live in buildings in crowded cities, who do not have this much luxury. Sometimes, going outside for them could be uncomfortable. Humans need sunlight, and in this chapter, we will discuss the benefits of going outside, especially on a sunny day.

Day 91 – Getting Outside Can Boost the Body's Vitamin D Supply

Did you know that vitamin D deficiency is usually caused by lack of sun exposure? The easiest way to get vitamin D is through bathing in the sun! Vitamin D is synthesized in the skin through a photosynthetic reaction triggered by exposure to ultraviolet B (UVB) radiation. Yes, you may take vitamin D supplements as well, but sunlight is free and natural. It's how humans are supposed to boost vitamin D supply – naturally from the sun.

If you have a chance to go outside, please do (with proper precautions, of course).[111]

Day 92 – Getting Outside Can Help with Bone Development

Aside from calcium and magnesium, did you know that vitamin D also plays a role in bone development? The following will be full of scientific terms, pardon me, but I need to explain it as accurately as possible.

The initial product of photosynthesis in the skin is Vitamin D3, and most of this is transformed into 25-hydroxyvitamin D, or Vitamin 25(OH)D. Vitamin 25(OH)D is then transformed to Vitamin 1,25(OH)D in the kidney. Vitamin 1,25(OH)D then enhances the absorption of calcium and phosphorus in the intestine. It also controls the flow of calcium into and out of bones to regulate bone-calcium metabolism.

Hence, prolonged vitamin D deficiency can make our bones weaker. Get outside and score some free Vitamin D![112]

Day 93 – Getting Outside May Prevent Rickets

As I have discussed in the previous benefit, vitamin D is needed in bone development alongside calcium. Extreme vitamin D deficiency can cause rickets in children. Rickets is a skeletal disorder wherein the bones become weak and soft. Do not be overly alarmed. As I've mentioned, it can only happen in extreme cases.

Children should regularly go outside because bone development is very crucial at their age. Tell your children that the sunlight helps absorb calcium and they would not grow properly without sunlight![113]

Day 94 – Getting Outside May Help Treat Tuberculosis (TB)

Tuberculosis (TB) is now curable, thanks to the discovery of streptomycin by Selman Waksman in 1943. Aside from the effective medical treatments, did you know that sun exposure can also help treat tuberculosis? Studies show that high vitamin D levels can reduce the risk of active TB by as much as 32%. That's a pretty huge risk reduction, and we can enjoy that for free through regular sun exposure![114]

Day 95 – Getting Outside May Decrease the Risk of Developing Multiple Sclerosis (MS)

Some evidence suggest that high levels of vitamin D may decrease the risk of developing multiple sclerosis (MS), a serious disease of the central nervous system that has no cure. While the cause of MS is unknown, one of the risk factors is having low levels of vitamin D because of low sunlight exposure.

According to statistics, there are nearly 1 million people who are affected by the disease in the United States. We don't want to be one of them. The cost of treatment is very expensive. Let's harness the power of sunlight and prevent many diseases from developing. Go outside![115]

Day 96 – Getting Outside May Lower the Risk of Developing Type 1 Diabetes

If you have type 1 diabetes, your body does not produce insulin, and you will be dependent on taking insulin for the rest of your life. Did you know that your vitamin D levels can greatly affect your chances of developing this disease? Studies show that vitamin D could lower the risk of developing type 1 diabetes by as much as 80%, while lack of vitamin D could increase the risk four times as much.

Do you still not want to go outside and let sunlight touch your skin?[116]

Day 97 – Getting Outside Can Prevent Hypertension

Hypertension has many risk factors, and most of them can be avoided, like smoking, being overweight or obese, being physically inactive, eating too much salt, and drinking too much alcohol.

High vitamin D levels, which could be achieved by enjoying the sunlight, can normalize blood pressure. Take a walk, enjoy the sun, and breathe fresh air. Sometimes we need some time alone and it's best if we spend it with nature.[117]

Day 98 – Getting Outside Can Prevent Cardiovascular Disease

Did you know that patients with cardiovascular disease are often found to be deficient of vitamin D? We discussed in the previous page that hypertension can be treated with vitamin D. Well, hypertension is one of the leading risk factors of cardiovascular disease. Therefore, lack of vitamin D can increase your risk of developing the disease.

As we grow old, we should be more physically active to maintain good stamina. One thing we can do is to walk for at least 30 minutes per day under the morning sun.[118]

Day 99 – Getting Outside Can Lower the Risk of Developing Prostate Cancer

According to research, men who are vitamin D deficient have an increased risk of developing prostate cancer. If you already have prostate cancer, the vitamin D analogue (modified form of vitamin D) *1a,24-dihydroxyvitamin D2* (1,24-[OH] 2D2) can stop its growth.

Today, many men rarely go outside because they are engaged in playing video games. Not only that, but they are also not physically active. They are unable to generate vitamin D naturally because sunlight does not touch their skin. If you're one of these people, I hope you take some time to go outside at least twice a week, or even better, make it every day if you can.[119; 120]

Day 100 – Getting Outside Can Lower the Risk of Developing Colon Cancer

One of the risk factors of colon cancer is being physically inactive. It is indeed more comfortable to just sit on the couch and watch TV. If we understand the underlying risks of being physically inactive, like the risk for colon cancer, I think it could give us some fear and motivation to exercise and be physically fit.

Research shows that patients who are newly diagnosed with colon cancer are vitamin D deficient. Vitamin D repletion is even recommended during chemotherapy. Get outside in the sun and give yourself the chance to avoid developing colon cancer.[121; 122]

Day 101 – Getting Outside May Protect Against Rheumatoid Arthritis

While there are available medications for treating rheumatoid arthritis, did you know that it has no cure?

Research shows that vitamin D deficiency is highly prevalent among patients with rheumatoid arthritis. Being overweight can also increase the risk of developing rheumatoid arthritis. Maintaining a healthy weight by controlling our food intake and exercising regularly may help protect against the development of rheumatoid arthritis. Going for a walk in the sunlight can have a great impact on your health![123]

Day 102 – Getting Outside Can Help Alleviate Asthma

Nowadays, asthma is more manageable than ever, but it still brings a lot of discomfort. If you have asthma, you may be cautious of your environment, and you need to have an inhaler wherever you go.

Studies have found that vitamin D deficiency is a cause, if not the leading cause, of the global asthma epidemic. In asthma management, Vitamin D is proven to be effective in combination with prescribed medications.

If you can find a place where you can bathe in the sun without triggering your asthma, take advantage. Take a walk for at least 15 minutes in the morning. The vitamin D that your body will generate can be beneficial to your condition.[124]

Day 103 – Getting Outside May Inhibit Induction of Systemic Lupus Erythematosus

Systemic lupus erythematosus, or lupus for short, is an autoimmune disease wherein the immune system attacks healthy tissues by mistake. One of the factors that can increase the risk of having the disease is vitamin D deficiency. If you already have lupus, studies show that ample levels of vitamin D can help you by inhibiting the activity of the disease. However, excess sun exposure can trigger the symptoms, so limit the time you go outside, and you can also try vitamin D supplements to bring you relief. Check with your doctor about what is safe for your situation.[125; 126]

Day 104 – Getting Outside May Inhibit Induction of Inflammatory Bowel Disease

Inflammatory bowel disease happens when you have inflammation in your digestive tract. According to studies, vitamin D promotes anti-inflammatory T-cells and cytokines, the deficiency of which is associated with increased disease activity, inflammation, and relapse. In other words, vitamin D can provide relief, but the treatments advised by the physician should be prioritized for immediate recovery.[127]

Day 105 – Getting Outside Could Inhibit Induction of Thyroiditis

Studies show that patients with hypothyroidism also suffers from vitamin D and calcium deficiency. It is recommended for these patients to be supplemented with vitamin D to help with the treatment, alongside the lifelong intake of levothyroxine (synthetic thyroid hormone) or other hormone therapies. If you have this disease, take advantage of the sun to produce your own natural vitamin D.[128]

Day 106 – Getting Outside May Increase Sperm Motility in Men

Aside from the quality and volume of sperm cells, their movement, or motility, is also important. Normally, sperm cells need to move at least 25 micrometers per second to conceive. Studies show that vitamin D may increase sperm motility by increasing the adenosine triphosphate (ATP) concentration which is important to generate sufficient force to overcome physical barriers in the female tract.

If you are trying to conceive, don't just stay at home and watch TV. Take some time to walk or jog in the park to increase your Vitamin D.[129; 130]

Day 107 – Getting Outside Could Inhibit Induction of Lyme Arthritis

Lyme disease is caused by a bacterium called Borrelia, which is spread by bites from infected ticks. The primary treatment is antibiotics for immediate recovery. Aside from that, patients with this disease are observed to have low vitamin D levels. Increasing these levels either by supplements or sunlight is important because of the anti-inflammatory properties of Vitamin D. This boost in Vitamin D levels may help inhibit the induction of Lyme Arthritis.[131]

Day 108 – Getting Outside Can Promote Better Sleep

If we have trouble sleeping, it is possible that our vitamin D levels are low. Vitamin D deficiency is observed to increase the risk of sleep disorders. Though it needs further investigation, initial studies show that vitamin D could help in the prevention and treatment of sleep disorders as the vitamin D receptors are widely distributed in the human brain, such as the hypothalamus, prefrontal cortex, midbrain central gray, substantia nigra, and raphe nuclei, all of which are known to execute important roles in sleep regulation.

Exercising in the morning can also help you sleep better at night. If you take a long walk or jog outside to start your day, you will not just be getting benefits from the exercise itself, but from the morning sun as well. Not only c̄ you improve your blood circulation, you can also get some of the vitamin D that your body needs every day.[132; 133]

Day 109 – Getting Outside May Help in Losing Weight

Did you know that exposure to sunlight can help you lose weight? Studies show that light exposure during the daytime can influence body weight regardless of sleep timing and duration. It can also decrease the risk of developing obesity.

While you're at it, why not do some exercise under the sun in the morning? Losing weight needs dedication and constant motivation. Understanding the health benefits of being physically fit will give us more reason to do so.[134]

Day 110 – Getting Outside May Link to Longer Life

In the previous pages we discussed health benefits of sun exposure and vitamin D, and it's quite obvious that it can help us live longer. Avoiding the aforementioned diseases gives you a more comfortable and less stressful life ahead.

Aside from this, there are studies showing that those who spent more time under the sun lived six months to two years longer than those who had less sun exposure. It may not sound that long, but two years is still two more years to spend with your loved ones.[135]

Day 111 – Getting Outside May Help Treat Psoriasis

About 2.2% of the US population is affected with psoriasis. It's a skin disorder that is itchy and painful. It's not a deadly disease, but it brings discomfort and may affect self-confidence because it's not pleasing to the eyes.

If you have this disease, sunlight can be your friend. Sunlight can help slow down skin growth through its UVB rays. Moreover, studies show that low vitamin D levels worsen the disease while increasing vitamin D levels reduces its severity.[136]

Day 112 – Getting Outside May Help Treat Eczema

There are at least 30 million people in the US who suffer from eczema, a condition wherein the skin becomes itchy, scaly, and inflamed. If you have this disease, sunlight may help ease the symptoms through vitamin D, which controls the local inflammatory immune response. However, too much sunlight can worsen the symptoms, so you must not stay outside for too long. If your condition is severe, taking Vitamin D supplements is more recommended than direct sun exposure to avoid flare ups caused by too much heat from the sun.[137]

Day 113 – Getting Outside May Help Treat Jaundice

A person with jaundice may have unusually yellow skin and eyes due to high levels of bilirubin, a yellowish pigment that is excreted from the liver which is responsible for the yellow color of urine and the brown color of feces. The jaundice itself is not dangerous, but the underlying conditions might be, such as hepatitis, gallstones, and pancreatic tumor. Also, it has been observed that patients with jaundice have significantly lower vitamin D levels as compared to those who do not have the disease. If you have jaundice, it can help if sunlight touches your skin every day to produce ample amounts of vitamin D.[138; 139]

Day 114 – Getting Outside May Help Prevent Acne

Almost all of us have suffered from acne at least once in our lives. There are people who frequently have it resulting in a loss of self-confidence. Studies show that patients with acne are frequently vitamin D deficient, and lower vitamin D levels could worsen the skin condition.

Sunlight can worsen acne, but it may prevent it from happening if you consistently have enough vitamin D in your body. While your skin is still smooth, let sunlight touch your skin, especially in the morning.[140; 141]

Day 115 – Getting Outside Can Reduce the Risk of Seasonal Affective Disorder (SAD)

Seasonal affective disorder (SAD) is a type of depression that happens in a particular period or season of the year. One of the probable causes of this is low serotonin levels in the body. When you stay indoors for too long, it could mean less exposure to sunlight, which in turn could lower your serotonin levels, all of which can increase the risk of having seasonal affective disorder.

If you live in a place where the winter is usually hard, then it may be very uncomfortable or perhaps dangerous at times to go outside. In that case, there are available treatments and medications, but you should consult a doctor first for correct prescription.[142]

Day 116 – Getting Outside May Prevent Overeating

Did you know that sunlight may prevent us from overeating? Studies show that eating in a dark environment may trigger the appetite and make you want to eat more. Therefore, it may be better to open the windows and drapes and allow sunlight to enter the house while eating. You should also avoid eating late at night, or what we call "midnight snacking." Instead of basking in the glow of your refrigerator light, get outside and enjoy your meal al fresco![143]

Day 117 – Getting Outside May Maintain the Efficiency of the Eyes

If you have children, make sure to inform them of this. Studies show that children who are exposed to more sunlight have reduced risk of developing nearsightedness. It is very important not to give children total freedom in using their electronic gadgets, especially late at night. Encourage them to play outside and be exposed to sunlight. Children need to be physically active for their bone and muscle development, and the sunlight can also help their eyesight.[144; 145]

Day 118 – Getting Outside May Help as Part of Liver Cirrhosis Treatment

Studies show that patients with cirrhosis who are vitamin D deficient have increased risk of mortality and infections. While further studies are needed to determine its pathogenic association with advanced liver fibrosis, some studies suggest that sufficient levels of vitamin D promotes higher virological response to treatment. In other words, patients with cirrhosis can benefit from vitamin D, which can be produced by the body through sunlight exposure.

There are about 4.5 million adults in the US who are diagnosed with cirrhosis, and one of the causes of cirrhosis is alcohol abuse. Always remember that alcohol can damage the liver. Your liver needs to function properly if you want to live a long life.[146]

Day 119 – Getting Outside May Help in Thrombosis Treatment

Thrombosis happens when the blood clots within a blood vessel, which disturbs the normal circulation of blood. Studies show that vitamin D can be potentially effective in preventing thrombotic disorders caused by hypoxia, or lack of oxygen in the tissues.

If you are diagnosed with thrombosis, moving frequently may help speed up recovery to get your blood circulating more. Take a walk in the park when you can, breathe fresh air, and feel the warmth of the morning sun.[147]

Day 120 – Getting Outside May Help as Part of Irritable Bowel Syndrome Treatment

Studies show that serotonin (a hormone that may increase upon sun exposure) is one of the main factors in maintaining gut motility, which may help in treating irritable bowel syndrome (IBS). Serotonin has many other benefits, such as keeping you from experiencing mood swings, anxiety, and depression.

Take the opportunity to be sun-kissed every now and then if you suffer from IBS. Patients with IBS are also advised to exercise regularly, so it would be best to do it every morning when the sunlight is not too hot.[148]

Key Takeaways

We may have been focusing on eating healthy foods so much that we have forgotten the health benefits of sunlight and the danger of not being exposed to it. If you have read the entire chapter, it should give you more reason to go outside and not just stay at home whenever you're free.

Maintaining sufficient vitamin D levels is not too hard. Sunlight is free for us to benefit from every single day. The funny thing is that some people make sure that their plants are well-sunlit but not themselves. They don't realize that their bodies need sunlight, too.

If you live in a country with long winters and you need to stay inside for months, I suggest taking vitamins, including but not limited to vitamin D, to at least compensate for the missed benefits of sunlight. Remember to eat healthy foods, too, because some people take vitamins but continue to eat unhealthy foods, mistakenly thinking that the vitamins will save them from diseases.

Do not forget that too much sun exposure can also cause health problems, such as skin cancer. If you know that you are going to be exposed to the sun for longer periods of time, apply sunscreen to be safe.

Vitamin D deficiency is not a joke. It can bring many health complications, so always take some time to go outside, even for just 15 minutes a day.

Month 5 – Grounding

In the modern times, wearing footwear such as slippers, sandals, and shoes is common, even inside our homes. Our reasons could be dirty floors, comfortability, or we just don't want to step on things that could injure us. These are good reasons, but we could be missing out on something that is extremely important to our health.

This chapter will focus on grounding, or earthing. You may not have heard about this, but it is simply connecting to the Earth's surface and reaping tons of health benefits through its vast supply of free electrons. We will discuss the benefits of walking barefoot, and I hope to change your mind about wearing footwear all the time.[149]

If you forgot to purchase your grounding mat, that's okay! Get one as soon as possible, but keep reading so you don't break your daily habit!

Day 121 – Grounding May Promote Better Sleep

Grounding is not just done by walking barefoot. There are products available to do grounding even while sleeping, such as conductive carbon fiber mattress pads (which are connected to the ground). Studies have shown those who use these pads while sleeping have significantly improved the quality of their sleep.

If you are having trouble sleeping, this could be an option for you. The products are not that expensive, and you can use them for a lifetime, making this a good investment for your health. Not being able to sleep well can negatively affect your physical and mental performance, which you don't want to happen when you need to work.[150]

Day 122 – Grounding May Help Reduce Pain in General

We experience body pains as we grow older. We easily get tired, and our bones become weaker, especially if we do not regularly exercise. Even after a good sleep, we can still feel some pains in different parts of our body, like joints in the arms, knees, and hips.

Studies show that those who sleep while grounded (using grounding mats) experience less pain upon waking up. This is just one of the many wonders of being connected to Earth![151]

Day 123 – Grounding May Decrease Fatigue

Working all day can give us stress and fatigue, whether it be a physically or mentally exhausting job. The only hope we have for being able to work the next day is a good night's sleep.

Studies have shown that grounding while sleeping not only can decrease fatigue, but it can also increase your energy for the next day. Imagine waking up full of energy and ready to take on the world. We all want that![152]

Day 124 – Grounding Can Improve Mood

All of us can be moody at times. It usually happens when we are stressed or if we have problems that we overthink. People have different ways to improve their mood, like relaxing, meditating, going for a walk, or watching TV. Did you know that grounding can also improve your mood?

Studies show that grounding, even for only one hour, can significantly improve the mood as compared to just relaxing without grounding. This means that grounding can affect our bodies in a good way without any side effects.[153; 154]

Day 125 – Grounding Could Help Relieve Hypertension

If you have hypertension, the first thing you should do is avoid the things that can worsen your blood pressure, like eating salty foods. Hypertension is manageable, but should not be ignored, as it could lead to more serious health problems.

Grounding can help relieve hypertension. Studies show that hypertensive patients can significantly benefit from grounding if done at least ten hours per day for several months. This can be easily achieved if you avail a grounding mattress pad so you are grounded while sleeping.[155]

Day 126 – Grounding May Reduce Inflammation

Inflammation is your body's way of telling you that a foreign object has entered it and is not welcome. It attacks those foreign bodies and heals you in the process. While inflammation is a natural occurrence, chronic inflammation can increase the risk of developing various diseases.

Grounding can help manage inflammation. Studies show that grounding can significantly reduce inflammation by being grounded while sleeping even for at least four nights. Greater benefits against inflammation can be gained if done continuously for several weeks or months.[156]

Day 127 – Grounding Can Improve Circulation

Poor blood circulation can be caused by a variety of things such as by being obese or by having diabetes. If you have these conditions, grounding may help you improve your circulation. Studies show that grounding for at least 20 minutes can improve blood circulation and relieve symptoms like numbness of limbs, drying of skin, and hair fall, among others

Aside from grounding, regular exercise can significantly improve blood circulation. Exercises like jumping jacks or jogging in place can be conveniently done at home and do not require a lot of space. Maybe you could do these exercises outside and benefit from grounding AND get your sunlight to improve your Vitamin D?[157]

Day 128 – Grounding May Promote Better Cell Repair/Healing

Cell damage, or cell injury, happens when a cell suffers from stress which may or may not be reversible. It has many causes, such as lack of oxygen (hypoxia) or lack of adenosine triphosphate (ATP), both of which are essential for the cells to survive. Grounding can aid the body in repairing the damaged cells, allowing for them to continue with their normal functions.[158; 159]

Day 129 – Grounding Can Detoxify Your Body

Toxins can build up in the body by drinking too much alcohol, not getting enough sleep, not drinking enough water, eating foods high in sugar and salt, and many others. Detoxification is needed to get rid of toxic substances in the body. While our liver and kidneys naturally detoxify our bodies, some activities may help in detoxification, such as fasting and grounding. Even if you can help your body to detoxify, you should avoid altogether the aforementioned factors of toxin build-up. Prevention is still better than cure.[160]; [161]

Day 130 – Grounding Can Improve Immune Response

If your job exposes you to harmful substances, like working in a hospital, it is important to maintain a healthy immune system at all times. Grounding can improve the immune response to injury and infection, which gives better defense against bacteria, viruses, and other harmful substances.[162]

Day 131 – Grounding Can Restore the Body's Natural State

Did you know that grounding can help with jet lag? Stepping barefoot on the ground can restore the body's natural or normal state. Ease your jet lag with 30 minutes of grounding and you will be able to sleep better.[163]

Day 132 – Grounding Can Help with Arrhythmia

Regular grounding is known to help with inflammation. Since arrhythmia can be aggravated by inflammation, grounding may help patients with arrhythmia. Still, prescribed medications should be prioritized for immediate relief. Consult a doctor right away if the symptoms are unbearable.[164]

Day 133 – Grounding May Reduce Muscle Pain and Damage After Exercise

Studies have shown that grounding can significantly decrease muscle damage after exercise by reducing the creatine kinase loss from the injured muscles.

If you are already outside, take off your shoes and put your feet on the ground for several minutes. Just relax for a while and let your body heal through grounding.[165]

Day 134 – Grounding Can Slow Down Aging

Grounding is known to have anti-aging effects by neutralizing excess free radicals in the body. Free radicals can help protect your body from pathogens, but too many can be damaging. It can cause diseases such as diabetes and cancer.

If you want to get optimum anti-aging results, your diet should consist of foods high in nutrients and antioxidants, plus regular exercise should be part of your routine. Also, stop smoking and limit alcohol intake. Not only will our physical appearance look younger, but our organs will also function properly, which is essential to a long lifespan.[166]

Day 135 – Grounding Might Reduce Body Voltage

Having static electricity is usually not dangerous, but it can be annoying at times. It can make your hair stand up, and you can get zapped when touching people or objects, which hurts quite a bit. Grounding can be effective in reducing the electric fields induced on the body. The electrical potential of the body and the Earth can equalize through the transfer of electrons between them.

Take note that static electricity can damage electronic components, so before touching any delicate electronics such as circuit boards, make sure you do not have static charge buildup.[167]

Day 136 – Grounding May Reduce Osteoporosis

Grounding is found to have positive effects in osteoporosis. When grounded, the concentration of minerals such as calcium in the blood serum can improve by reducing the renal excretion of calcium. Therefore, the risk of developing osteoporosis can be reduced.

Osteoporosis usually happens after age 50, when the bones start to break down more than they form. Even if you are not yet 50 or older, take some time to do grounding to get its benefits on your bones. It's free, harmless, and very easy to do![168]

Day 137 – Grounding May Promote Better Digestion

Grounding is found to aid digestion through thermal imaging technology. During grounding, a patient is observed to have better blood circulation, which prevents bloating and congestion in the digestive tract.

Still, the best way to have better digestion is to eat foods high in fiber. This is discussed in "The Beauty of Good Carbs" chapter.[169]

Day 138 – Grounding Can Relieve Asthma

Grounding can help people with asthma by relieving inflammation. With constant grounding (especially during sleep), the use of inhalers and other medications can be lessened as asthma attacks can be significantly reduced. If you have asthma, give grounding a chance and observe its positive effects on your body. Grounding does not have any known side effects with asthma, so do it as much as you can.[170]

Day 139 – Grounding May Improve Focus

Conscious grounding can help improve your focus and concentration. Stand on the ground barefoot, or if you cannot stand, sit on a chair. Incorporate meditation while grounding and focus on the present moment. (See the "Meditate" chapter later in this book for more information). Your blood can begin to circulate better to your brain, which can improve your concentration. Do this for at least half an hour to gain its benefits.[171]

Day 140 – Grounding May Prevent Anxiety

High cortisol levels are linked to anxiety. When you feel anxious, your cortisol level can shoot up. Grounding can help regulate the cortisol levels and can ease anxiety.

Aside from treatments, we must also help ourselves determine the things that make us anxious and work to find relief. Anxiety is no joke, and it can greatly affect our daily lives. Take advantage of the health benefits of grounding and ease your anxiety in the process.[172]

Day 141 – Grounding Can Promote Weight Loss

Grounding is found to be beneficial to people suffering from obesity. It can promote better digestion and blood circulation, which can help ease many discomforts in obese people.

If you really want to lose weight, grounding is just one of the many things that you should do. The weight loss journey can be long and difficult, but with constant exercise, it can turn into habit, and you'll be fit eventually. Believe in the process and do not expect changes to happen overnight.[173]

Day 142 – Grounding Can Help Prevent Cancer

Cancer may develop with high concentrations of free radicals in the body. Grounding is known to neutralize these free radicals, hence lowering the risk of developing cancer.

There are many ways to prevent the development of any type of cancer, but there is no guarantee that we won't develop one. Be that as it may, we should always be mindful of what we eat and of our overall lifestyle. This book has tons of useful information that could change your life around, so keep on reading and let us all promote optimal health![174]

Day 143 – Grounding May Prevent Multiple Sclerosis (MS)

Multiple sclerosis (MS) is a serious medical condition with no cure, though there are several therapies that could help ease the pain. One of those therapies is grounding. Inflammation is one of the signs of MS, and grounding can be an effective anti-inflammatory therapy.[175]

Day 144 – Grounding May Reduce Lupus-Related Pain

Lupus is an autoimmune disease which attacks the body's own tissues and organs. It has no cure, but there are available treatments to manage it.

Various studies have shown that grounding can reduce pain in patients suffering from lupus, as well as other autoimmune disorders. Connecting oneself to the ground is also observed to be very beneficial to the immune system through Earth's limitless supply of mobile electrons. Without mobile electrons, the body will be more vulnerable to diseases.[176]

Day 145 – Grounding May Prevent Inflammatory Bowel Disease (IBD)

Inflammatory bowel disease is characterized by chronic inflammation of the digestive tract. Long-term grounding may help ease the pain caused by the IBD, since grounding is shown to be effective against inflammation.

Doctors may prescribe anti-inflammatory drugs, and that's fine, but you don't want to be heavily dependent on these drugs because of their side effects. Grounding, on the other hand, only offers positive effects on the body.

To get the benefits of grounding sooner, try grounding mats so you can sleep while grounded. Do this continually for a few days and you may already notice the relief. Do this for weeks and then several months and I am confident that you will feel a lot better.[177]

Day 146 – Grounding May Help Patients with Diabetes

According to studies, continuous grounding can significantly decrease blood glucose in patients with diabetes. This is good news because diabetes has no cure and grounding is extremely easy to do.[178]

Day 147 – Grounding May Prevent Rheumatoid Arthritis

Grounding may prevent the development of rheumatoid arthritis by hindering the immune system from attacking the cartilage in joints. Like lupus, rheumatoid arthritis is an autoimmune disease that has no cure, but treatments are available to make it manageable.

Grounding is a free and safe way to boost the immune system. Before buying various vitamins, consider grounding first.[179]

Day 148 – Grounding May Prevent Uveitis

Uveitis is an inflammation of the uvea, the vascular middle layer of the eye. It requires immediate treatment for the patient to recover or else it could cause blindness.

Grounding is proven to be effective in reducing inflammation in various parts of the body, and it could help prevent uveitis as well. While the exact cause of uveitis is unclear, you can reduce the risk by constant grounding.

Again, uveitis requires immediate treatment and grounding is only for prevention. Grounding does not treat uveitis.[180]

Day 149 – Grounding May Help Prevent Glaucoma

Glaucoma is a common eye condition, especially for older people. Some of the risk factors are obesity and high blood pressure. Since grounding is beneficial against both conditions, it may lessen the risk of developing glaucoma.

While further studies are required to determine the effects of grounding to the eyes, grounding remains safe and effective in keeping our bodies healthy.[181]

Day 150 – Grounding May Increase Heart Rate Variability

Grounding is generally beneficial to the heart by increasing the heart rate variability (HRV). Studies found that people who have high HRV have healthier hearts, and healthy hearts can adapt more to the environment and be more resilient to stress.

Next to the brain, the heart is one of the primary organs that keep us alive. Keeping it healthy will also keep the other organs functioning properly. On top of grounding, you must be physically active as well, and stay away from greasy foods as much as possible.[182]

Key Takeaways

Grounding is an overlooked therapy with all the modernizations around us. We tend to lean towards medications right away, not even considering the natural ways of healing the body. Have a headache? Take an aspirin. Have a common cold? Take dextromethorphan. But have you ever even thought about grounding?

The human body's components can all be found on the Earth. Even without understanding the science behind grounding yet, it is not absurd to think that stepping barefoot on the ground can have positive effects on the body.

In fact, it was observed that the advent of footwear with insulating soles in the 1950s has led to the increase of diseases worldwide. Though there is no hard evidence, it is logical to conclude that these kinds of footwear took the immune system by surprise. Earth is the body's primary source of electrons, and insulated footwear has deprived the body of electrons.

Humans are meant to connect to the Earth. Traditional leathers are fine, but modern shoe styles typically have rubber soles. Yes, they are more comfortable and more flexible, but they don't connect us to the Earth like humans used to do.

I hope you have learned the health benefits of grounding in this chapter. It's free and very easy to do. Grounding products are also not that expensive, and you can use them for years until they wear out. Let us all promote a healthier life through grounding!

Hello!

Before you get started with Month 6, this is a reminder that you will need to purchase magnesium for your new daily habit beginning in Month 7. Although we will mention magnesium spray in Month 7, if you chose to use a dietary supplement for your magnesium instead, that is perfectly fine. If you have questions about which type of magnesium will work best for you, feel free to reach out to your doctor or another trusted health professional before making a purchase.

A special note: We will be discussing ashwagandha in Month 8. If it is easier to purchase your supplements at the same time, consider buying your ashwagandha now as well.

Okay, you may continue to improve your health now!

Month 6 – Park on the Farthest Side of the Parking Lot

You might ask, "Why would I park on the farthest side of the parking lot? What am I, crazy?"

Hear me out first. Walking is dreaded by many. With the advent of cars, bikes, and scooters, who would want to walk for miles? While it is much more convenient and faster to ride, many of us tend to abuse getting on wheels. Vehicles have become cheaper as well. There are now also compact variants of cars if you are on a tight budget.

This is bad news. Did you know that more than 40% of the US population is obese? This is roughly 131 million individuals. While this is mainly caused by the generally unhealthy American diet, this is also caused by lack of exercise.

In this chapter, I will remind you how walking is important to our health. You brought your car? Park on the farthest side of the parking lot![183]

Day 151 – Walking Can Improve Blood Circulation

Walking is one of the simplest exercises that can get your heart rate up, which can help improve your blood circulation. Studies show that simply walking for at least 30 minutes a day can reduce the risk of stroke by 20%. Powerwalking could reduce it even more by 40%!

In the US, someone dies from stroke every four minutes. We could change that data if we just exercise more and eat healthier foods. Remember that we are not getting any younger. Let's improve our lifestyle before it's too late.[184]

Day 152 – Helps Protect Against Loss of Bone Mass

Bone loss starts to occur at the age of 30. Regular walking can prevent, or at least slow down, the loss of bone mass. Your diet can also significantly affect your bones. Eating foods high in calcium, such as dairy and green leafy vegetables, can help protect your bones.

Back in the day, people were used to walking for miles frequently because transportation was not always available. If you're going to a place that is just a couple of miles away, consider walking unless it's dangerous or very inconvenient. Take the opportunity to use your feet to get you to your destination once in a while.[185]

Day 153 – Walking Can Help Prolong Life

Research shows that people in their 50s and above who walk regularly are less likely to die in the next eight years. You see, being physically inactive can bring many health problems. You can easily get fat because you don't burn the calories you eat. You can develop heart disease early in life if you don't move enough.

If you are already 50 years old and above and do not have much to do, I urge you to exercise regularly, unless you can't exercise due to health reasons. Being old does not mean you should stay at home all the time. If you can walk or jog, do it every day. Just don't overexert yourself to prevent too much stress to your heart.[186; 187]

Day 154 – Walking Can Improve Mood

Have you ever felt like going on a long walk when you were stressed? That is because walking releases endorphins that can relieve stress and pain. Whenever you're bummed out, take a walk and it can literally improve your mood. While walking, you can take the opportunity to think as well.[188; 189]

Day 155 – Walking Can Help with Weight Loss

Walking frequently can help you lose weight. Try brisk walking or powerwalking and it will burn even more calories. If walking has become too simple for you, maybe you can put on some ankle weights to add some challenge. Wrist weights are also available to help build muscles on your arms and burn fat.[190]

Day 156 – Walking May Help Strengthen Leg and Abdominal Muscles

Walking can strengthen the leg and abdominal muscles, especially when walking over elevations. If you're always walking on flat surfaces, try walking uphill for a change. If you're the adventurous type, you can try mountain hiking, but please do your research first if you don't have any experience yet. Mountain hiking is fun and challenging, but it could be dangerous depending on the trail.[191; 192]

Day 157 – Walking May Help You Sleep Better

In a study of 59 people with an average age of 49.43 (±8.40) years, results show that participants had better sleep quality (but not duration) when they were made to walk daily for four weeks. There are many reasons why a person can't sleep, but if the body is tired during the day, the body would want to rest more. If you're just resting all day, you will find it hard to sleep at nighttime.[193; 194]

Day 158 – Walking May Help to Keep Your Joints Strong

When you walk, you move the joints in your ankles, knees, hips, and shoulders, among others. Any movement that you do helps to lubricate the joints, which can decrease pain, especially for people with arthritis. It is important that you keep moving not only for your joints, but also for your muscles and bones. You can also do some stretching upon waking up to remain flexible and prevent possible injuries.[195; 196]

Day 159 – Walking May Boost Your Energy

Many of us drink coffee in the morning to give us a boost of energy. Did you know that walking may be a better option for giving you an energy boost than caffeine? This was observed in a study participated in by young women aged 18 to 23 years who were sleep deprived. Instead of giving them caffeine, they were made to walk on the stairs, and their energy exceeded those who took caffeine.[197; 198]

Day 160 – Walking Can Help Improve Memory

Are you becoming forgetful? Be more active! Studies show that people who are more physically active develop better memory than those who are less active. Don't just stay at home and watch TV. Take a walk in the park and make some sweat![199]

Day 161 – Walking Can Lower the Risk of Having Alzheimer's

In a study that was participated in by men whose ages were between 71 and 93, results show that those who walked more than a quarter mile every day cut the incidence of dementia and Alzheimer's disease in half. Can you believe it? This is just walking not for even more than a mile every day, and it can already save you from a dreaded disease.[200]

Day 162 – Walking May Help Lower Blood Sugar

A small study showed that having a 15-minute walk after every meal is more effective in lowering blood sugar than taking a one-time 45-minute walk. If you have high blood sugar, you may want to consider this. Yes, it requires some effort, but it's for your own benefit. Plus, walking offers many other benefits, so it's only a win for you.[201]

Day 163 – Walking May Help Boost the Immune System

A study was made during a flu season wherein 1,000 participants were made to walk 30 to 45 minutes per day. Results showed that not only did they have fewer sick days, but the symptoms were also lessened. If you're worried about getting sick because you have many responsibilities, consider walking for at least 30 minutes a day. Believe me, it will pay off.[202]

Day 164 – Walking May Help Boost Creative Thinking

Research shows that walking is very effective for increasing creativity, especially in those who walk outside rather than walking on a treadmill. Walking outside provides you with sunlight, the benefits of which are discussed in the chapter "Get Outside." Moreover, you'll be able to breathe fresh air, unless your environment is heavily polluted. In that case, you may want to find a place with cleaner air to walk in.[203]

Day 165 – Walking Can Delay the Appearance of Varicose Veins

As we age, varicose veins will appear more if we're not physically active. Not only do they look unsightly, but they are also painful. Walking can delay the appearance of varicose veins as it allows your blood to flow properly. If your job is to sit all day, take some time to walk before or after your work shift to improve blood circulation.[204]

Day 166 – Walking Can Improve Bowel Movements

Walking is obviously effective on your leg muscles, but it can also be effective in strengthening the muscles in the abdomen, which promotes better movement in the gastrointestinal tract. Constipated? Don't just rely on medicines. Take a walk for at least 10 minutes each day and it can help you recover from constipation.[205]

Day 167 – Walking May Counteract the Effect of Obesity-Promoting Genes

Research shows that brisk walking for at least 30 minutes a day could cut the effects of obesity-promoting genes in half. If your family has a history of obesity, you could become obese, too, if you're not careful. Take a walk every day and improve your lifestyle. Stay away from fatty and sugary foods to avoid developing obesity. If you can do more than just walking, all the better! Take a jog or do sprints to burn more calories.[206]

Day 168 – Walking May Reduce the Cravings for Sweets

For those who have a sweet tooth, walking for at least 15 minutes could help reduce your cravings for sweet foods. If you do not limit yourself in eating sweets, it can bring many health problems, such as diabetes, heart disease, liver disease, and tooth decay. Sometimes it's just hard to refrain from eating your favorite foods (which are usually unhealthy), but you should always remember the effects of those foods on your health. Eat sweet foods in moderation.[207]

Day 169 – Walking May Reduce the Risk of Developing Breast Cancer

Research shows that walking for at least seven hours a week could reduce the risk of developing breast cancer. This is just one hour a day. While most breast cancers develop at age 50, you should not wait to reach that age to exercise. Take some time to walk, preferably early in the morning to also get the benefits of sunlight. Remember that prevention is better than cure.[208]

Day 170 – Walking May Reduce the Risk of Developing Colon Cancer

Research shows that people who are physically active are less likely to develop colon cancer. Like breast cancer, most colon cancers develop at age 50 or older. This gives us more reason to be physically active, and walking is one of the easiest exercises we can do.[209]

Day 171 – Walking Can Help You Sweat

Walking, especially power walking, can make you sweat. There are many potential benefits of sweating, such as better blood circulation, release of toxins and salts, and bacteria reduction on the skin. If you live in a cold climate, wear sweaters or thick clothes while walking to help your body sweat more. Don't hesitate to sweat, it's good for you.[210]

Day 172 – Walking Can Help You Increase and Maintain Flexibility

People who do not exercise regularly can find it difficult to move because their joints become stiff due to lack of exercise. Flexibility, or the range of motion that your joints can move, can be increased by walking. Stretching before and after walking is recommended for better flexibility and less possibility of injury.[211]

Day 173 – Walking Can Help Prevent Hip Fracture

Being more physically active is required as we grow older to strengthen our muscles and bones. Walking could increase bone density in the legs, thus reducing the risk of hip fracture.

A 30-minute walk in the park per day would be enough, but if you can do longer, all the better. Drink lots of water to keep you hydrated. Refrain from walking under intense heat as it could induce hypertension, which is common in older people.[212]

Day 174 – Walking Can Be Safe for People with Exercise-Induced Asthma

Since walking does not require a lot of effort, it is an exercise that can be recommended for asthma patients. However, you should be careful of your environment. Do not walk when the weather is cold because cold, dry air could worsen asthma. A warm and humid environment is most suitable for walking for asthma patients.[213]

Day 175 – Walking Can Give You More Money!

We normally prefer convenience, and truth be told, convenience has a cost. For example, instead of walking to a destination that is only one or two miles away, some would choose to bring their cars, even if it's not really needed.

Walking can be the cheapest option to get to your destination, and I urge you to walk instead of ride. Not only is it free, but you will also reap the benefits of walking.[214]

Day 176 – Walking Can Help with Lower Back Pain

Research shows that walking regularly can reduce lower back pain. If your job makes you sit for hours, sometimes it's difficult to maintain a proper posture, which could result in back pain. Walking allows you to use many of your joints and improve flexibility.[215]

Day 177 – Walking Can Promote Better Eyesight

People who are physically active can have healthier eyes and a reduced risk of developing retinal problems. Instead of spending hours upon hours watching TV or using the computer, take care of your eyes and go outside. Engage with people so that you will not be bored in doing physical activities.[216]

Day 178 – Walking Can Prevent Brain Shrinkage

Research shows that older people who walk for at least six miles per week can prevent or slow down brain shrinkage. Not only is walking beneficial to the bones of older people, but it can also be beneficial for their brains. If you cannot walk that far, do some other exercises at home which you are more comfortable with to maintain good blood circulation.[217]

Day 179 – Walking Can Keep You Motivated

Brisk walking for at least 30 minutes in the morning could give you an energy boost and motivation lasting throughout the day, according to studies. Before drinking your favorite morning beverage, go outside and exercise. Take advantage of morning sunlight for your body to generate vitamin D and perspire at the same time. It may give you not only motivation all day, but it could also make it easier for you to sleep at night.[218]

Day 180 – Walking May Lower the Risk of Miscarriages

Walking in the morning can be healthy for pregnant women, unless it is strictly advised by the doctor to have complete bed rest. If your pregnancy is perfectly healthy, do not be afraid to walk. Walking can reduce stress hormone levels, which helps lessen the risk for miscarriage as well.[219]

Key Takeaways

Walking is one of the easiest exercises, but sadly many people are still too lazy to walk. People have become too reliant on the modern transportation options available, and they choose to ride even if their destinations are just two miles away. As a result, people have become more prone to diseases. They become fatter because they don't burn enough calories.

I know that it's a lot more convenient to ride a vehicle, but walking is needed by our bodies to be healthy. Decades ago, humans walked more, and obesity was not a common disease. Today, just look around. Many people have become fat because of modern transportation, not to mention the processed foods and sugary drinks. If you continue this lifestyle, it's just a matter of time before you develop a disease and cut your life by many years.

Having said these things, I strongly urge you to walk as much as possible. Walking under the morning sun is a better option to benefit from vitamin D. Brisk and power walking will yield better results.

Let us not wait to have a disease before we decide to exercise and maintain a healthy lifestyle. We only live once, so let's take our health seriously and enjoy the life we have been gifted.

Hello!

It's time for another purchase reminder! Month 8 will deal with ashwagandha, and now is a great time to purchase this supplement if you haven't already. Ask a doctor for advice if you are not sure where to start. As of the writing of this book, ashwagandha supplements are available for purchase through online retailers, including Amazon.

Let's get into Month 7!

Month 7 – Keep Magnesium Spray in the Shower

You've likely heard about magnesium and how important it is to the body. There is a good chance that you don't know all the things that it does, or how easy it can be to supplement the magnesium that comes in through your food.

While it is estimated that few people are significantly deficient in magnesium, those same studies show that the majority of people are not getting enough. Inadequate magnesium can lead to a wide variety of side effects. Magnesium plays a role in everything from metabolism to cellular generation, and even protein synthesis. Inadequate magnesium levels can contribute to diabetes, cardiovascular disease, and even osteoporosis. You'll see over the next month how important it is to your health.

There are a number of ways that you can supplement magnesium, but I have found the simplest one to be through the skin. You can purchase magnesium spray in a lot of places, which is both inexpensive and quickly absorbed. The best time I have found to use it is in the shower. It's right there next to the other products that I use, and quickly became part of my ritual. This is a great way to help create a healthy habit of using magnesium spray.

I suggest spraying it under your arms primarily, but you can spray it pretty much anywhere that there isn't hair. I don't have much on the top of my head, so I apply some there, too. I would strongly urge you to be careful of spraying it into your eyes, nose, mouth, or anywhere … below the waist.[220]

If you forgot to purchase your magnesium, that's okay! Buy it as soon as you can, but keep reading so you don't break your daily habit!

Day 181 – You Can Replenish Your Magnesium Level Quickly

In the introduction to magnesium, we talked about the fact that we are recommending transdermal (through the skin) magnesium rather than through food. You might be wondering why?

Generally, getting your needed minerals through food is the best way. I would love to be able to tell you that this would be adequate, but unfortunately, with commercial agriculture and food processing, we aren't getting as much magnesium as we should be. This is why so many people are lacking proper levels of magnesium.

Yes, you can take a magnesium supplement as a pill or even a drink. I am the first to admit that there are institutional cautions on taking transdermal magnesium, as there is question over the effectiveness. However, both the research that I've done myself and the benefits that I have received personally suggest to me that it is worthwhile. If you prefer to consume a pill, powder, or other injectable form of magnesium, I won't fault you for it.[221; 222]

Day 182 – Magnesium May Relieve Stress

If you take a look at many of the current crop of stress reduction pills, creams, and gummies, you'll find many of them have magnesium as an ingredient. Why? It's because magnesium deficiency often leads to anxiety and stress symptoms. While there are other reasons you might feel stressed or anxious, applying magnesium when you're in the shower may help.[223]

Day 183 – Magnesium Can Relieve Muscle Cramps

Muscle cramps are an interesting phenomenon. People experience them at a variety of different times and for different reasons. Some of the reasons include mineral deficiencies, and magnesium deficiency can be one of them. If you suffer from muscle cramps, topical magnesium spray in the shower may help reduce them.[224; 225]

Day 184 – Magnesium May Prevent Fatigue

Magnesium is essential to quite a few biological processes, and magnesium deficiency can result in a wide variety of symptoms. One of these symptoms is fatigue. Modern life is tiring, and some people believe that we can't find relief from that exhaustion, but it's just not true. One of the likely ways to combat fatigue is to make sure your magnesium levels are adequate. The next time you take a shower, be sure to spray yourself a few times with your topical magnesium spray.[226]

Day 185 – Magnesium May Treat Chronic Pain

Increasing your magnesium intake may reduce pain. Magnesium blocks the *N-methyl-d-aspartate* (NMDA) receptor channels in the spinal cord, limiting the influx of calcium, which may reduce the risk of excitotoxicity, which in turn can lead to oxidative stress, neuronal cell death, and excessive stimulation of receptors. If you don't experience chronic pain, that's a great thing, but it doesn't mean you won't see benefit from using magnesium spray.[227]

Day 186 – Magnesium May Prevent Tremors

Similar to the potential benefit of relieving cramps is the benefit of reducing or even preventing muscle tremors. Notice that there are a variety of relaxation benefits from magnesium – cramps, anxiety, and now tremors. When the body is balanced and operating well, many of the symptoms of modern life can fall away. This may all contribute to a more relaxed way of life, with fewer or even no muscle tremors. Take your magnesium![228]

Day 187 – Magnesium May Prevent Irregular Heartbeat

We have this theme running with magnesium, about how it may have significant impact with muscle function. Well, your heart is a muscle, so it's probably no surprise that magnesium may have an impact on your heart. Magnesium has been shown to positively impact arrythmia or irregular heartbeat. If this is a condition you already experience, you likely have a treatment plan. For the rest of us, this is just good information to have. That magnesium you spray on in the shower may be benefitting all of your muscles, including your heart.[229]

Day 188 – Magnesium May Prevent Migraine

It's hard to be able to know how many people experience migraine headache symptoms, as the data varies wildly, but there's a good chance that you'll experience a migraine at some point in your life, if you haven't already. Migraines can be reduced or even eliminated when magnesium levels are brought in line.

Low magnesium levels may cause abnormal glutamatergic neurotransmission which showed in many neurological and psychiatric disorders such as migraine. This is why some migraine supplements and medical protocols include magnesium. Spray away![230]

Day 189 – Magnesium Can Help Alleviate Anxiety and Depression

Ever feel anxious or depressed? A lot of people do. As you've already read, magnesium may help with those feelings. I've personally experienced benefit with my symptoms of anxiety from daily magnesium intake, but your results may vary. Some studies even claim magnesium as a critical component in preventing depression. Magnesium modulates glutamatergic neurotransmission which may prevent the feelings of stress and anxiety. Even if you're not chronically stressed or anxious, spraying magnesium on in the shower can help with the more challenging days we experience.[231; 232]

Day 190 – Magnesium May Prevent High Blood Pressure

We all know that high blood pressure is something to avoid, and magnesium levels can have an impact. A lack of magnesium may cause an increased concentration of intracellular calcium which narrows the blood vessels. (Another example of a tissue relaxing when magnesium levels are appropriate!). Whether you're showering today or not, spray some magnesium on your body.[233]

Day 191 – Magnesium Can Prevent a Heart Attack

Similar to the impact on blood pressure by opening up blood vessels, magnesium can impact your heart. Proper magnesium levels can keep the heart working properly and can reduce the risk of heart complications.[234; 235]

Day 192 – Magnesium Can Prevent Stroke

According to statistics, someone in the US has a stroke every 40 seconds, while someone dies from it every four minutes! This is an alarming number of people suffering from stroke. Unhealthy diet is the main contributor to the disease as more and more people prefer processed foods over vegetables and manually cooked meals.

Magnesium can play an important role in preventing the development of stroke. While a healthy diet should be the number one priority, magnesium intake or topical application can be helpful in preventing the disease. Remember that stroke can lead to death if not treated immediately, not to mention the high cost of treatments. Like they say, prevention is better than cure, so buy your magnesium now![236]

Day 193 – Magnesium May Help Prevent Dementia

When we grow old, we don't want to forget our children and our loved ones. We also don't want our children to suffer taking care of us. Sadly, over 6 million Americans are affected by the disease and 1 out of 3 seniors dies with dementia.

Studies show that ample magnesium levels in the body can decrease the risk of developing dementia by 30%. There's a warning – very high levels of magnesium can increase the risk of dementia as well. It's better to check your magnesium levels with lab tests at least annually along with your general check-up.[237]

Day 194 – Magnesium Can Prevent the Progression of Chronic Kidney Disease (CKD)

Did you know that about 37 million people are suffering from chronic kidney disease in the US alone? This is a staggering number which we should be alarmed of since this could cause an early death for many people.

Normal magnesium levels in the body can help prevent chronic kidney disease by preventing mineral buildup in the blood vessels due to phosphate overload.[238]

Day 195 – Magnesium Can Prevent Hearing Loss

Magnesium can also play a role in our hearing. As we already know, hearing declines with old age, but we can still do something to prevent it. Magnesium can increase the blood flow in the cochlea, a part of our ear which has a significant function in hearing, which can prevent and limit hearing loss.[239]

Day 196 – Magnesium Can Promote Healthy Pregnancy

If you're pregnant, you will do your very best to stay healthy for your baby. You will eat healthy foods, take supplements, get enough sleep, and exercise as well. You must also know that magnesium can be very important in preventing complications in pregnancy.

Before taking magnesium supplements or applying transdermal magnesium, ask your doctor first for advice on whether you need a prescription. Women have different bodies and diets after all, so you may or may not need the extra magnesium. Always remember to be very careful of what you eat and take during pregnancy.[240; 241]

Day 197 – Magnesium Can Promote Better Lactation

Being a mother to a baby is stressful. You will always have to be vigilant so you may not get enough sleep even if you want to. As a result, your stress levels may go up which could affect your milk supply and contents. Magnesium can promote better lactation by relieving your body of stress.[242]

Day 198 – Magnesium May Treat Asthma

Asthma has different severities, but all asthma patients can encounter severe asthma attacks. Magnesium sulfate (not just magnesium) is one of the medications that can be administered for severe asthma. It provides relief from symptoms by relaxing the bronchial muscles and expanding the airways to allow more air in the lungs. I know that this is different from magnesium sprays, but this explains how beneficial magnesium can be.[243; 244]

Day 199 – Magnesium May Help Prevent Osteoporosis

There are about 10 million adults in the US who are suffering from osteoporosis. This bone disorder inhibits patients from doing many physical activities as bones can break easily, and broken bones are painful.

One of the possible causes of osteoporosis is magnesium deficiency. Did you know that about 60% of magnesium is stored in the bone? Low magnesium levels in the body can impair bone growth and can make our bones fragile. Thus, sufficient levels of magnesium can prevent osteoporosis.[245; 246]

Day 200 – Magnesium May Help Treat Acid Reflux

If you are acidic, you have to be very picky about what you eat because some foods aggravate acid reflux. Oftentimes, people use antacids to relieve the pain, but did you know that magnesium can help with acid reflux as well?

Magnesium, when combined with hydroxide or carbonate ions, may help neutralize the acid in your stomach. One example of this is the milk of magnesia that can give short-term relief from acid reflux symptoms.[247]

Day 201 – Magnesium May Prevent Bloating

Bloating is not really a disease, but it can be uncomfortable at times. We usually bloat when we eat fast or if we chew gum, but aside from these there are many other factors that can contribute to bloating.

Magnesium can help with bloating, so if you feel bloated, quickly apply magnesium spray. Observe if the bloating goes away after some time. You may also drink a magnesium supplement for faster reaction since the bloating happens in the digestive tract.[248]

Day 202 – Magnesium May Prevent Insomnia

Have you experienced going to bed early, but you just can't fall asleep? Many people suffer from insomnia or sleeplessness. As a result, their productivity during the day is greatly affected, not to mention the health implications of not having enough sleep.

Magnesium can affect the body by activating the parasympathetic nervous system, which is responsible for the body's rest. If you find it hard to sleep, try spraying magnesium or taking magnesium supplements. Adequate levels of magnesium in the body can prevent sleep disorders.[249]

Day 203 – Magnesium Can Be Effective in Treating Premenstrual Syndrome (PMS)

While I may not be in the position to describe premenstrual syndrome, I know that it affects many of the female population, and that it is one of the hardest things about being a woman.

The good news is that there are ways to prevent it from happening, such as having a healthy lifestyle. Plus, magnesium, when combined with Vitamin B6, is proven to be effective in decreasing the symptoms of PMS. Studies show that the positive effects of magnesium will be experienced after at least two months of magnesium administration.

This is just one of the many benefits of magnesium, so don't forget to spray it on your body today![250]

Day 204 – Magnesium May Relieve Constipation

All of us may have experienced constipation even once in our lives, and it can be very uncomfortable. If you have constipation, you can buy over-the-counter medicines such as magnesium citrate to soften the stool.

Having the right amount of magnesium in the body constantly can alleviate the symptoms of constipation, so you'll have no regrets spraying magnesium on your skin daily.[251]

Day 205 – Magnesium Can Be Good for the Eyes

While we should take care of all our organs, we tend to neglect our eye health. Having bad eyesight makes you rely on your eyeglasses or contact lenses, and wearing them can be uncomfortable. Well, if you have the money, you can have Lasik surgery, but consider magnesium instead.

The good news is that magnesium can be extremely beneficial for eye health as it regulates cellular functions. Even patients with eye diseases such as glaucoma have shown great improvement just after four weeks of magnesium treatment.

Are you still hesitant to purchase a magnesium spray? My advice is to buy one now and reap the benefits of magnesium![252]

Day 206 – Magnesium Can Be Good for the Teeth

Dental health is as important as eye health. We use our teeth to grind our food, and of course, we'll look better and feel more confident when we smile.

Magnesium plays a role in the absorption of calcium. Even if the body has a lot of calcium, if it is magnesium deficient, calcium may not be absorbed properly by the body. Keep your teeth healthy and spray your magnesium on your body![253; 254]

Day 207 – Magnesium Can Prevent Nausea

Nausea can be caused by many things including magnesium deficiency. Magnesium has tons of contributions in the body such as blood glucose control, energy production, and normal heart rhythm. Having a magnesium deficiency in the body can cause nausea. Make sure your magnesium levels are maintained by spraying magnesium daily.[255; 256]

Day 208 – Magnesium May Prevent Seizures

There are many causes of seizures, and one of them is epilepsy. About one percent of the US population suffers from a form of epilepsy. While this is not a huge percentage and the seizures are usually manageable, it is still better to have our health in an optimal condition.

Studies have shown that magnesium deficiency contributes to the condition of patients who have seizures. Maintaining the magnesium levels for those patients has improved their condition, if not totally eliminated seizures.

As you see, not having enough magnesium in the body can cause a lot of health problems. Do not risk your health. Spray your magnesium instead![257]

Day 209 – Magnesium May Lower the Risk of Diabetes

About 10% of the US population has diabetes, and one of the factors of the disease is prolonged magnesium deficiency. Magnesium plays a role in glucose metabolism, so not having enough magnesium in the body can shoot up the blood glucose and worsen insulin resistance altogether.

If you are a diabetes patient, it is important to have your magnesium levels in check. Buy magnesium spray and apply it daily to ensure that your body gets the magnesium it needs.[258]

Day 210 – Magnesium May Help in the Treatment of Urinary Tract Infections (UTI) in Women

Urinary tract infection is prevalent in women because of their anatomy. Their urethras are shorter than men's, so bacteria can easily travel to the bladder. The good news is that magnesium intake (not the spray) is used in UTI treatment because it relaxes the smooth muscle of the bladder that helps inhibit frequent urination.

While the spray variant of magnesium is not used in the treatment, it is still important to maintain the right magnesium levels in the body.[259]

Key Takeaways

Did you know that about half of the US population is magnesium deficient? We know very well that many of us resort to processed foods because they are easy to prepare, and let's admit it, they're tasty as well. However, these processed foods do not give us the nutrition that we need and that includes magnesium. We need at least 300mg to 500mg of magnesium every day. As we have discussed in this chapter, there could be many health complications if we remain magnesium deficient for a prolonged period of time.

Magnesium helps with calcium absorption, that's why low magnesium levels correlate with low bone density. No matter how consistently we take calcium, it will not be absorbed by the body if we don't have enough magnesium. Magnesium is also responsible for the metabolism of vitamin D that our bodies generate when we go out in the sun. Vitamin D also plays a role in absorbing calcium. You can just imagine how magnesium is important for bone health.

Just a warning though, there are also health implications if we take too much magnesium. It could cause dizziness, blurred vision, and breathing difficulty. Be sure to follow the recommended dose of magnesium, whether the oral or the transdermal varieties.

Hello!

Month 8 is about to begin, and I hope you are feeling healthier already!

When we reach Month 9, we will be discussing Blue Blocker Glasses. If you would like to purchase yours to have them for the start of Month 9, now is a great time to shop. A health care professional may be able to guide you if you are not sure what to look for when shopping for blue blocker glasses. I was able to find blue blockers in a search on Amazon, so they are readily available and convenient to purchase.

Now, let's get back to improving your health!

Month 8 – Ashwagandha

Ashwagandha, sometimes referred to as Indian ginseng, is a medicinal plant with many proven health benefits. However, it's not in the same genus as ginseng. Ginseng is a root plant, while ashwagandha is a shrub that grows in India, the Middle East, and some parts of Africa. Even so, ashwagandha has tons of health benefits which we will discuss in this chapter. If you haven't heard about ashwagandha before, you'll be surprised how it can aid our health!

IMPORTANT: Not everyone responds to ashwagandha in the same way. You MUST speak with a health care provider before using ashwagandha.

If you forgot to purchase your ashwagandha, that's okay! Get it as soon as possible, but keep reading so you don't break your daily habit!

Day 211 – Ashwagandha Can Inhibit Tumor Growth

The first health benefit that I'll be telling you is that ashwagandha can inhibit the growth of tumors. Research studies show that ashwagandha has anti-cancer properties, and it can even reduce the side effects of anti-cancer agents. Therefore, ashwagandha is proven to be very helpful for cancer patients in their recovery. Moreover, long-term treatment using ashwagandha is also proven to be effective in treating fibroid tumors (or myomas).[260]; [261]; [262]

Day 212 – Ashwagandha Can Reduce Inflammation

Ashwagandha is effective against inflammation, according to studies. To expound, ashwagandha could inhibit an enzyme called *cyclooxygenase-2 (COX-2)*. This enzyme is responsible for the formation of *prostanoids* that consists of *prostaglandins*, which are vasodilators (widens blood vessels) that are involved in the inflammation process. In a nutshell, ashwagandha can help to narrow your blood vessels to prevent further inflammation.

If you're suffering from a disease that involves inflammation such as asthma and arthritis, you might want to consider taking ashwagandha supplements. It may be quite pricey depending on where you live, but you will feel its anti-inflammatory properties with continuous intake. Of course, you should prioritize taking medications prescribed by your doctor before taking anything else. Consult first your doctor if you would like to try ashwagandha.[263]

Day 213 – Ashwagandha May Have Antibacterial Properties

Animal and in vitro studies show that withaferin A (a natural product derived from ashwagandha) demonstrates antibacterial effects against *Staphylococcus aureus* (commonly found on people's skin), *Listeria monocytogenes* (commonly found in moist environments), *Bacillus anthracis* (commonly found in soil, water, and vegetation), *Bacillus subtilis* (commonly found in soil and in the gastrointestinal tract of ruminants and humans), *Salmonella enterica* (commonly found in the intestines of humans, animals, and birds), and *Salmonella typhimurium* (commonly found in raw or undercooked meat and eggs).

Taking ashwagandha could give you added protection against these bacteria. Of course, proper hygiene and cooking your food well can significantly lower the likelihood of bacterial infections.[264]

Day 214 – Ashwagandha Can Help Prevent Iron Deficiency Anemia

Ashwagandha has a natural iron content and has a positive effect on *hematopoiesis*, or the formation of the four blood cellular components: red blood cells, white blood cells, plasma, and platelets. If you are suffering from iron deficiency, you can also take an ashwagandha supplement on top of your iron supplement to potentially benefit from ashwagandha's many wonderful health effects.[265]

Day 215 – Ashwagandha Can Help Reduce Stress and Anxiety

When you are stressed, the circulating cortisol (stress hormone) in your body is elevated. Ashwagandha can substantially reduce the cortisol levels. Excess amounts of cortisol can result in increased *allostatic load* (or the wear and tear of the body), contributing to anxiety.

There are many things that can cause us stress, like deadlines and huge responsibilities. Ashwagandha can help your body cope with the stress that you experience regularly.[266]; [267]; [268]

Day 216 – Ashwagandha May Help Treat Schizophrenia

In a study involving 64 schizophrenia patients, their symptoms were reduced when they were administered ashwagandha (500 mg in first week and 1000 mg for the remaining 11 weeks).

If you are taking care of a schizophrenic patient, ask a doctor first about the dosage of ashwagandha that can be safely administered to the patient. Avoid giving a dosage based on what you just see on the internet or on TV because each patient is different and therefore could react differently to medications.[269]

Day 217 – Ashwagandha Can Help Reduce Food Cravings

Chronic stress may lead to increased food intake (or what we call stress eating), and since ashwagandha lowers cortisol levels, it can also help reduce food cravings. Remember that if you keep on eating excessively, not only could you become overweight, but you could also develop health complications such as heart disease and diabetes.

If you find it hard to control your eating habits, you may consult a dietician to give you expert advice on what you should eat. You may also consult a psychologist if you think your bad eating habits are caused by a psychological problem.[270]

Day 218 – Ashwagandha May Help Treat Alzheimer's Disease

Withaferin A, a natural component found in ashwagandha, is one of the *withanolides* that are beneficial in the treatment of Alzheimer's disease. However, please consult a doctor first before giving ashwagandha to a patient with Alzheimer's. While it has many proven health benefits, it could cause side effects when taken in large doses.[271]

Day 219 – Ashwagandha May Help Increase Muscle Mass and Strength

According to a study, a group of young men who had undergone resistance training, had greater increases in muscle strength and muscle mass when they were treated with ashwagandha. If you are trying to get in shape, then I highly recommend ashwagandha for you! Also, do not forget to have proper diet and complete sleep.[272]

Day 220 – Ashwagandha May Help Treat Diabetes

Withaferin A, which is found in ashwagandha, was found to increase glucose uptake, which means that it can be beneficial in treating diabetes. Consult your doctor first if you are interested in using ashwagandha for your diabetes treatment, so that your health can be monitored accurately along the way.[273]

Day 221 – Ashwagandha May Help Improve Semen Quality

A study showed that men who were treated with ashwagandha demonstrated increased semen quality which resulted in pregnancy for 14% of the patients. Sperm production may also improve due to ashwagandha's stress-reducing properties.

Ashwagandha is a safe supplement that you can take if you and your wife are trying to get pregnant. Before trying the expensive options, give ashwagandha a chance to help you conceive. Be sure to check with your doctor first.[274; 275; 276]

Day 222 – Ashwagandha Can Help Increase Testosterone Levels

According to a study that consisted of 57 men, their testosterone levels increased by 14.7% when they were treated with ashwagandha. Why would you want to increase your testosterone? The male hormone helps in building muscles, greater libido, and better erection. If you're a woman, ashwagandha is proven to be useful in the treatment of female sexual dysfunction (FSD) as well.[277]

Day 223 – Ashwagandha May Help Lower Cholesterol

A study performed in rats showed significant decrease in cholesterol when root powder of ashwagandha was included in their diet. While this is only an animal study, this could also have the same effect in humans.

Remember that the first and foremost solution in lowering cholesterol is by refraining from eating foods high in cholesterol. Simultaneously, take the medications prescribed by your doctor. Ashwagandha is generally safe so you can take it anytime, but if you have doubts, feel free to consult your doctor before taking.[278]

Day 224 – Ashwagandha May Improve Overall Brain Function

In a study that was conducted with 20 healthy male participants in which ashwagandha was administered to them, significant improvements were observed in brain tests such as simple reaction, choice discrimination, digit symbol substitution, digit vigilance, and card sorting tests.

If you are preparing for a big test or a job interview, you may take ashwagandha as this is observed to improve brain function. About the dosage, follow what is on the package and do not overdose.[279]; [280]; [281]

Day 225 – Ashwagandha May Improve Sleep Quality

In a study involving sleep-deprived rats, it showed that ashwagandha decreased cellular stress and cell death on a group of rats that was fed with ashwagandha for 15 consecutive days. This may only be an animal study, but this could have the same effect in humans as well. Try taking ashwagandha for 15 consecutive days or more and observe your sleep quality.

Remember that there are many factors that can affect your sleep quality. You should be aware of those factors first before acting on them. If your sleep quality is affected by anxiety, then you should work on your anxiety as well. Ashwagandha may help, but it's not the cure.[282]

Day 226 – Ashwagandha May Increase Swimming Performance

A study was done in mice in which they demonstrated a significant increase in swimming time when they were treated with ashwagandha. As you may have read in the previous pages, ashwagandha has anti-stress properties which could help a person to achieve more physically and mentally. Take ashwagandha if you want to improve your endurance and overall performance in whichever physical activity you are into.[283]

Day 227 – Ashwagandha Could Prevent Stress-Induced Ulcers

A study performed in rats indicated that ashwagandha was effective in stress-induced gastric ulcers. A 15-day treatment significantly reduced secretion of gastric juices and total acidity.

If you are frequently stressed about many things, ashwagandha may help you manage your stress. Do not ignore stress. Prolonged stress can cause many serious health problems, including heart disease.[284; 285]

Day 228 – Ashwagandha May Reduce Leukocytosis

Leukocytosis, or the increase in white cell count in the blood that is higher than normal range, was reduced by ashwagandha treatment in a study performed in mice. If you have this disease, you must prioritize the treatments advised by your doctor before taking ashwagandha. Remember that ashwagandha is just a supplement that can help you recover, but not the primary treatment.[286]

Day 229 – Ashwagandha May Help Alleviate Depression

A study was performed on 64 adults undergoing stress and it showed a 79% reduction in severe depression. As you may know, stress can cause anxiety and depression. If you are depressed, you may not know yet exactly the cause of your depression, but there's a good chance that you are stressed as well. Working on your stress can significantly alleviate your depression, and ashwagandha can help.[287; 288]

Day 230 – Ashwagandha May Prevent Signs of Aging

Ongoing studies show that ashwagandha could delay aging by increasing the activity of *telomerase*, an enzyme that restores short bits of DNA called *telomeres*. As the cell divides recursively during mitosis, *telomeres* are shortened until the cell reaches the Hayflick limit, which is around 50-70 times before experiencing cellular senescence. *Telomerase* allows the cell line to divide without reaching the limit.

Pardon the scientific terms! You may research about these to learn more. The important takeaway is that ashwagandha can prevent the signs of aging, but remember not to do anything that could cause aging, such as smoking cigarettes and drinking alcohol.[289; 290]

Day 231 – Ashwagandha May Relieve Arthritis

In a study that was undergone by 125 patients with joint pain, their rheumatoid arthritis seemed to become better when they were treated with ashwagandha and *sidh makardhwaj*. However, further studies are required to verify these findings.

Please consult your doctor immediately if you have arthritis to get proper treatment. You may take ashwagandha on the side to help with the arthritis and to benefit from its other potential health effects.[291; 292]

Day 232 – Ashwagandha May Relieve Pain

Ashwagandha is also an analgesic that can relieve pain by preventing the pain signals from traveling the nervous system. However, this is not as quick and effective as actual painkillers, so if you're suffering from intense pain, ashwagandha is not the way to go. Consult your doctor for prescriptions if you are experiencing chronic pain. Take note that overdosage of painkillers can be lethal, so be mindful of how much you take and work as a partner with your doctor to develop your treatment plan.[293]

Day 233 – Ashwagandha May Help People with Bipolar Disorder

In a study, 53 bipolar patients showed improvement in auditory-verbal working memory, reaction time, and social cognition when treated with ashwagandha. However, further study is recommended for more concrete data.

Whether you have bipolar disorder 1 or 2, try taking ashwagandha and observe if the severity and frequency of your manic episodes will lessen.[294]

Day 234 – Ashwagandha May Help People Undergoing Chemotherapy Treatment

Ashwagandha can help patients with breast cancer in all stages who are undergoing chemotherapy treatment by relieving cancer-related fatigue.

If you are undergoing chemotherapy, tell your oncologist first if you will be taking ashwagandha so that he or she is aware. Remember to disclose everything you take to your doctor especially if you are trying to recover from a serious illness.[295]

Day 235 – Ashwagandha May Help People with Obsessive-Compulsive Disorder (OCD)

A study involving 30 patients with diagnosed OCD showed that ashwagandha may be beneficial to the treatment of OCD as a supplement.

In the prior pages I have mentioned that ashwagandha is beneficial to the brain's overall performance. The exact cause of OCD is still unknown, but current research suggests that it involves problems with communications in different parts of the brain. Therefore, ashwagandha may be helpful to OCD patients in some way.[296; 297]

Day 236 – Ashwagandha May Improve Running Performance

Ashwagandha may improve running performance by improving lower limb muscular strength and muscle memory. If you're a male, you may benefit from ashwagandha even more since it boosts the testosterone levels, which is beneficial to the muscles.[298; 299]

Day 237 – Ashwagandha May Reduce Fat in the Blood

Ashwagandha may lower triglyceride levels of patients with metabolic problems due to high triglyceride levels. People with normal triglyceride levels are not likely to be affected by this, so ashwagandha is still safe to take.

If you currently have high triglyceride levels, consult a doctor immediately, as it could lead to organ problems if not treated. Take ashwagandha only as a supplement and not as a primary means to normalize your triglyceride levels.[300]

Day 238 – Ashwagandha May Help Treat Dry Mouth

Since ashwagandha is *anxiolytic* (reduces anxiety), dry mouth that is caused by anxiety can be treated by ashwagandha supplementation.

If you currently have dry mouth and aren't sure of the cause, the best thing to do is to consult a doctor. Do not self-diagnose or self-medicate to avoid further complications.[301]

Day 239 – Ashwagandha May Boost Alertness

A small study was performed and ashwagandha demonstrated a positive effect on mental alertness with a proper dosage for at least 14 days.

This adds to the proof that ashwagandha supplementation promotes brain health. It has no side effects with a proper dosage, so you can enjoy its benefits without worrying.[302]

Day 240 – Ashwagandha May Improve the Overall Quality of Life

A study showed that ashwagandha can improve the overall quality of life. The participants in the study were treated with 600mg of ashwagandha for 12 weeks. The participants displayed improved physical function, psychological health, and social relationships, among others. No wonder ashwagandha has been used for thousands of years without any issues![303; 304]

Key Takeaways

Ashwagandha has been used as an herbal medicine for at least 6,000 years, according to historical records. It has tons of health benefits for the body, which encouraged many scientists around the world to investigate deeper on the plant. Many clinical studies were done both on animals and humans, and ashwagandha is proven to be effective in reducing stress, boosting testosterone, increasing muscle mass, lowering cholesterol, improving brain function, and many others. It is also generally safe to take, but you should always ask your doctor first if you have an existing illness. The rule of the thumb is when you are in doubt, ask for professional advice first. If you don't feel good after taking ashwagandha, refrain from taking it and immediately seek medical attention.

Ashwagandha supplements can be purchased from Amazon for less than $20 per bottle as of this writing. There are several brands available so you should read the reviews first before making the purchase.

Month 9 – Wear Blue Blockers (Light Timing)

When going to the beach or even just going out on a sunny day, some of us wear sunglasses to protect our eyes from ultraviolet rays and see better. Well, some wear it only for fashion, but it has an actual benefit to the eyes. Our eyes are sensitive and can be damaged easily. Wearing sunglasses is a cheap way to provide protection to our eyes.

Did you know that there is a different type of sunglasses that can give you more health benefits?

First, let's discuss blue light. Blue light is emitted from light-emitting diodes (LED) which are used in almost everything that produces light, such as phones, tablets, computer screens, household bulbs, car dashboards, and televisions. Blue light per se is not bad, but it can affect our brains through our eyes, so a type of sunglasses was developed to block the blue light. These special glasses are called blue blockers.

Learn the effects of blue light in this chapter and be surprised how blue blockers can make you healthier.

If you forgot to purchase your blue blocker glasses, that's okay! Get them as soon as possible, but keep reading so you don't break your daily habit!

Day 241 – Blue Blockers Can Help to Prevent the Body from Being Awake

Blue blockers are glasses with specially crafted lenses, typically with an orange tint, which block out blue light emitted from lighted electronics as well as other sources. Studies have proven that blue blockers can prevent light-induced melatonin suppression. Melatonin helps us sleep better, and it should not be suppressed at nighttime. Our biological clock is most sensitive to short wavelengths (blue light) and exposure to them will trick our brain into thinking that it is still daytime. This suppresses the release of melatonin, so we will not feel sleepy at bedtime.

Blue blockers are very recommended for people who work late at night to help them sleep more easily immediately after work.[305]

Day 242 – Blue Blockers May Promote Better Sleep

Aside from helping you get to sleep more easily, which we discussed in the previous benefit, wearing blue blockers whenever necessary can improve sleep quality. Bad sleep quality will make you feel tired in the morning even if you have slept for eight hours.

If you can prevent using gadgets or watching TV before sleeping, that would be ideal. If you can't avoid it due to all sorts of reasons, I recommend that you wear blue blockers to help you sleep better.[306]

Day 243 – Blue Blockers May Improve Overall Mood

There are times when we wake up still feeling tired, even if we have slept for 7-8 hours. As a result, we could be moody, and not just in the morning, but maybe for the entire day. The goal is to wake up feeling great without any headaches and fatigue, right?

Studies have shown that mood can be significantly improved by blue blockers by allowing the person to have better sleep quality.[307; 308]

Day 244 – Blue Blockers May Prevent Heart Disease

According to studies, sleep deprivation can increase the risk of developing coronary heart disease and dying from it. With blue blockers, you would be able to sleep easier even if you are frequently exposed to blue light.

Do not ignore sleep deprivation. You may tell yourself that you can survive up to three days without sleep. Yes, the human body can do that, but it's never okay. Our brains and organs need to rest or else our bodies will shut down.[309]

Day 245 – Blue Blockers May Reduce the Risk of Type 2 Diabetes

Studies have shown that better sleep quality can help prevent type 2 diabetes.

If you really want to prevent diabetes, eat healthy foods and have an active lifestyle. If you are currently overweight, you must work on it as soon as possible because it is a risk factor in developing the disease.[310]

Day 246 – Blue Blockers May Help Against Depression

People with depression may spend a lot of time looking at screens which emit blue light, resulting in a disturbed biological clock. While blue blockers are not a cure to depression, they can help improve sleep quality by not suppressing the melatonin production in the body.

If you have been diagnosed with depression, or if you believe you are depressed, it can be helpful to talk to people close to you, whether they are friends or family. Healthy social relationships can be one of the ways to alleviate depression. If you don't have anyone close to you that you feel comfortable approaching, you could speak with your doctor for some direction. There are also folks you can reach out to anonymously. Help is always out there, and you should never feel ashamed for trying to improve yourself.[311]

Day 247 – Blue Blockers May Help Against Anxiety

Anxiety can cause lack of sleep, and vice versa. Allowing your body to rest peacefully at night can reduce anxiety, which can be achieved by wearing blue blockers, allowing your body to release the melatonin that will help you sleep.

There is no exact treatment for anxiety, but you can help yourself overcome it. If it's already taking a toll on your daily life, I would advise seeking professional help soon. Psychologists are very good at helping you overcome anxiety.[312]

Day 248 – Blue Blockers May Help Treat Insomnia

People with insomnia usually take melatonin supplements to aid in their sleep. Since melatonin is produced by the body naturally with darkness, blue blockers can increase its production by simply blocking blue light.

You must treat your insomnia as soon as possible because it can greatly affect your daily life. Try wearing blue blockers and see if it helps you.[313]

Day 249 – Blue Blockers May Reduce the Risk of Obesity

In today's world, more and more people have access to gadgets which emit blue light from their screens. Exposure to blue light will make you feel awake, especially at night. It will disrupt your body clock resulting in sleep disorders, which in turn increases the risk of developing obesity.

Yes, sleep disorders can contribute to obesity, so don't just eat healthy foods and exercise. You also have to sleep![314]

Day 250 – Blue Blockers May Improve the Sleep Quality of Cataracts Patients

Studies have shown that blue blocker implants (not the one that is worn like sunglasses) can significantly improve the sleep quality of cataracts patients. If you have a cataract, you may suggest this to your ophthalmologist.[315]

Day 251 – Blue Blockers May Improve Memory

Many studies prove that sufficient proper sleep is beneficial to memory, especially when in stage four sleep (very deep sleep). That is why it is highly recommended that you sleep well before an exam.

If you notice that you have had bad memory recently, maybe you're not getting enough sleep. Try wearing blue blockers, especially at night, to help you sleep better.[316; 317]

Day 252 – Blue Blockers May Improve Concentration

Do you remember when you were in school, and you did not have enough sleep the previous night? It was difficult to listen to your teacher, right?

Studies show that a lack of sleep negatively affects concentration. It reduces your overall attention, and you will not be able to take in more information, so avoid driving (or any high-risk activities) when you do not have enough sleep![318]

Day 253 – Blue Blockers May Improve the Immune System

During sleep, small proteins called *cytokines* are released by the immune system. Enough sleep may increase the production of these *cytokines* which are crucial for fighting off infections.

Yes, having consistently good sleep is very beneficial for your immune system. You must sleep more if you are currently sick to help your body recover faster.[319]

Day 254 – Blue Blockers May Reduce the Risk of High Blood Pressure

The less you sleep, the higher your blood pressure can go. Getting to sleep on time can help you sleep for enough hours, thus reducing the risk of hypertension. Try wearing blue blockers if you find it hard to sleep at night.

However, sleeping completely is not enough to reduce the risk of hypertension. You have to be physically active and limit salt and fat intake. If possible, refrain from drinking alcohol as well.[320]

Day 255 – Blue Blockers May Improve Sex Drive

If you are always tired due to lack of sleep, your sex drive can be greatly affected. Lack of sleep can cause your body to suppress the production of sex hormones while the stress hormones go up.

This is one of the problems of busy couples. They are both very occupied, and when they are together in bed, they are both tired and do not have the drive to have sex. Try wearing blue blockers to help you have good quality sleep. In the morning, maybe you'll have the energy to have some "sexy time."[321]

Day 256 – Blue Blockers May Improve Balance and Coordination

According to studies, sleep deprivation impairs cognitive and motor performance with the same effect as legally prescribed (moderate) levels of alcohol intake. If you are sober but sleep-deprived, you should NOT drive. It's very risky. Work on improving your sleep to help save not only your own life, but perhaps someone else's life as well.[322]

Day 257 – Blue Blockers May Promote Better Skin

Wondering why you have wrinkles at such a young age? Studies have shown that people who don't get enough sleep (less than or equal to 5 hours) have higher levels of transepidermal water loss (TEWL), which could result in those wrinkles. On the other hand, those who sleep seven to nine hours a day have a 30% greater skin barrier (after tape stripping during the experiment) and have significantly better recovery from *erythema* (superficial reddening of the skin, usually in patches) after sun exposure.[323; 324]

Day 258 – Blue Blockers May Reduce the Risk of Death

It is common knowledge that frequent sleep deprivation could result in serious health conditions. If prolonged, it could result in death. Let blue blockers help you have better sleep quality and duration.

I understand that some people need to work double shifts to pay for their rent and bills. Surviving is difficult nowadays. If you really need to stay awake, at least take vitamins and eat healthy foods to compensate for not being able to sleep completely.[325]

Day 259 – Blue Blockers May Help Prevent Bone Mass Reduction

Recent studies show that chronic sleep deprivation decreases the bone mineral density and levels of 25-hydroxyvitamin D, which helps the body to absorb calcium (see the chapter "Get outside"). Good sleep is recommended to maintain optimal bone health.[326]

Day 260 – Blue Blockers May Prevent Fatigue

Good sleep quality can allow your body to rest and recover from fatigue. If you are frequently not sleeping properly, it can result in fatigue, and you may not be able to function properly.

Having quality sleep is not enough to fully recover from fatigue. You also must be well-hydrated and physically active. Avoid the things that make you stressed if possible. Refrain from smoking and drinking alcohol. Instead, drink water or fruit juices and eat healthy foods.[327]

Day 261 – Blue Blockers Can Decrease the Risk of Accidents

Poor sleep quality can adversely affect your cognitive function which can result in poor attention, slow reaction, and poor decision-making. You must avoid doing high-risk activities when you are sleep deprived.

Many accidents have happened due to poor cognitive function. Losing your focus could result in serious accidents and death. Probably one of the most common types of accidents is road accidents. Driving requires 100% attention on the road, especially at high speeds. Blue blockers can help you improve your sleep quality, reducing the risk of these accidents.[328]

Day 262 – Blue Blockers May Increase Muscle Strength

Studies have shown that those who do not get enough sleep (less than six hours) have their muscle strength reduced while those who sleep for seven hours or more have greater muscle strength.

If you're aiming to build muscles, you must avoid staying up late at night. Wear blue blockers to potentially help you sleep better.[329]

Day 263 – Blue Blockers May Help with Chronic Pain

Recovering from illness requires constant good sleep. Studies have shown that sleep deprivation can lead to systemic inflammation, which aggravates pain. Also, long-term good quality sleep may improve the condition of people experiencing chronic pain.

Do not ignore being sleep-deprived because it can take a toll on your health. Wear your blue blockers and you may improve your sleep and overall health.[330]

Day 264 – Blue Blockers May Relieve Stress

While stress can affect sleep quality, insufficient sleep can also induce stress. Having enough sleep can help your body to recuperate from stress. Moreover, those who sleep during the day have higher cortisol (stress hormone) levels than those who sleep at night. If your job requires you to work at night, take vitamins and make sure that you rest well during the day, and don't forget to wear your blue blockers to potentially improve your quality of sleep.[331]

Day 265 – Blue Blockers May Decrease the Risk of Alzheimer's Disease

People with Alzheimer's disease are found to have large numbers of *amyloid plaques* and *neurofibrillary tangles*. *Amyloid plaques* are extracellular deposits of the *amyloid beta (Aβ) protein* which increases with lack of sleep.

Wear blue blockers to likely prevent sleep deprivation and decrease the risk of developing Alzheimer's disease in old age. It's cheap and effective![332]

Day 266 – Blue Blockers May Prevent Dental Problems

Studies show that lack of sleep can increase your risk of developing dental problems and gum infections. Sleeping for seven to eight hours every night can maintain good dental health, on top of recommended dental care. Blue blockers can help you improve your sleep quality, and they may help you fend off the scary parts of dental exams that we all dread.[333]

Day 267 – Blue Blockers May Decrease the Risk of Catching a Cold

Studies show that not having enough sleep will make you more susceptible to a cold because lack of sleep leads to a poorer immune system. When you are sleep deprived, chances are you'll catch a cold. Having enough rest, on the other hand, can protect you from infection. Wear your blue blockers and avoid that cold![334]

Day 268 – Blue Blockers May Decrease the Risk of Colorectal Cancer

Studies show that sleeping less than six hours daily can significantly increase your risk of developing colorectal adenomas, which can turn into cancer when not removed. Blue blockers can help improve your sleep and help you reduce your risk of colorectal cancer.

To further prevent colorectal adenomas, eat lots of fruits and vegetables to take care of your gut health.[335]

Day 269 – Blue Blockers May Decrease the Risk of Stroke

Even if you are still young, do not make it a habit to be sleep-deprived. One of the long-term effects of sleep loss is increased stroke risk, and stroke is deadly. Stroke commonly happens to older people, but it can occur in all age groups. Do not be careless with your health. Potentially prevent all sorts of diseases by wearing blue blockers and getting better sleep.[336]

Day 270 – Blue Blockers May Prevent Loss of Motivation

Waking up from only a few hours of sleep will leave you feeling tired, and it can even be accompanied by headache and fatigue. Not allowing your body to rest can affect your mood for the entire day, which can decrease your motivation to do your tasks.

Boost your motivation through good quality sleep, which can be achieved by wearing blue blockers hours before bedtime.[337]

Key Takeaways

Like our laptops and phones, our bodies need to recharge to go through another day. Sleeping is the best way to recover from fatigue, especially if you are physically and mentally drained during the day. Even if you are taking tons of supplements, having ample sleep is still required.

While sleep deprivation cannot always be avoided, like for those who are taking care of their babies, wearing blue blockers can help normalize the melatonin production, which helps you sleep easier. Mothers need these the most because when the baby wakes up, they also wake up.

Those who work during the night should wear blue blockers because their computers emit blue light. After work when it is already morning, they should continue wearing blue blockers until they get home to protect their eyes from blue light. It can be much easier to sleep because the melatonin production is not suppressed as much.

Wearing blue blockers does not take much of an effort, but it can be helpful in many ways, most especially for our sleep. It is also cheap, and you usually don't need to buy another pair unless they break. It is a good deal that you can't ignore!

Month 10 – Breathing

In this chapter, we'll discuss things about the most basic task that we do every day: breathing. Surprisingly, many people are not conscious of what they breathe. If they can breathe without any difficulties, that's enough for them, but that should not be the case. Like the food that we eat, we should also be conscious of the air that we breathe.

Industrialization has greatly increased air pollution worldwide. As of this writing, the most polluted city in the US is Los Angeles, which is also the second-most populated city next to New York. If you still don't know, heavily polluted air can cause a wide variety of diseases especially to the lungs. Sadly, we don't have much of a choice if we live in these kinds of cities.

That's why various organizations around the world promote tree planting to help combat pollution. If you don't have a backyard, you can buy plants in pots and put them inside your home. Snake plant is one of the most common house plants and their care is fairly simple. Moreover, snake plants can convert carbon dioxide (which we exhale) to oxygen (which we inhale) at night, thus it promotes healthy air in the house.

We will discuss the benefits of breathing fresh air and you will find that it's extremely important to breathe fresh air regularly.

Day 271 – Breathing Fresh Air May Promote Better Digestion

Did you know that breathing fresh air can affect our digestion? Yes! An ample supply of oxygen can help the body to digest food properly since the muscles along the digestive tract need oxygen to function effectively.[338]

Day 272 – Breathing Fresh Air Can Improve Blood Pressure

Breathing fresh air can also regulate blood pressure. One of the symptoms of low blood oxygen levels is high blood pressure. Breathing fresh air can help the blood pressure go back to normal levels from being too high or too low.[339]

Day 273 – Breathing Fresh Air May Improve Overall Mood

Studies show that a reduced supply of oxygen in the brain has adverse effects in mood states. Lack of oxygen can make you less social, think less clearly, and feel dizzier.

If you notice you're moody, try going to a park with lots of trees. Take a walk and just breathe. You may notice that you'll feel better, unless your mood swings are caused by something else, e.g., hormones. If enjoying the fresh air isn't providing relief, check in with your doctor.[340]

Day 274 – Breathing Fresh Air Can Strengthen the Immune System

Breathing fresh air is very beneficial to the immune system. Lack of oxygen could make the immune system overreact and attack itself. Cells need oxygen to survive. An ample supply of oxygen allows the immune system to function properly and protect you from infections, and that is protection we always need.[341]

Day 275 – Breathing Fresh Air Can Help You Have Healthier Lungs

Not surprisingly, our lungs are the first and foremost organ affected by the air that we breathe. Constant exposure to air pollution, even just cigarette smoke, can already be damaging to the lungs.

If you are a parent and you have a child at home, do not smoke cigarettes near your child, or other people for that matter. People who breathe secondhand smoke, even if they are non-smokers, can still develop asthma and other lung problems. Let us be responsible members of society and let's not affect other people's lives with of our vices.

For the non-smokers, feel free to go out for a walk or just sit in the open air if someone lights up a cigarette inside. It's perfectly acceptable to take necessary actions to protect your own health.[342]

Day 276 – Breathing Fresh Air Can Give You More Energy

Our body needs oxygen to convert the food we eat into energy through the process called cellular respiration. Without a sufficient supply of oxygen, our food may not be properly converted into the energy we need to function.

If you feel weak, maybe you are just not breathing enough oxygen. Open your windows or go outside and breathe some fresh air.[343]

Day 277 – Breathing Fresh Air May Boost Alertness

Not breathing enough oxygen could make you feel dizzy in just a few minutes. Our brain needs a constant supply of oxygen to function properly.

If you notice that you're not thinking straight, maybe you just need to breathe some fresh air. Go to places with trees and grass, and, most importantly, far from air pollution.[344]

Day 278 – Breathing Fresh Air May Reduce Dynamic Hyperinflation

An ample supply of oxygen can help reduce dynamic hyperinflation caused by exercise, anxiety, respiratory distress, and many others.

Dynamic hyperinflation can also occur in asthma patients during their spontaneous breathing episodes. If you have asthma, I advise you to breathe fresh air in places where you know there are no irritants. Always bring your inhaler with you in case of asthma attacks.[345]

Day 279 – Breathing Fresh Air Can Help Fight Obesity

Studies have shown that the air we breathe affects our weight. Pollution can disrupt our metabolism, though the effects can only be seen long-term. A large study was done over a 14-year period, and it was observed that the people who lived in heavily polluted areas had hypertension and increased waist circumference as compared to those who lived in areas with generally fresh air.[346; 347]

Day 280 – Breathing Fresh Air Can Reduce the Risk of Inhaling Airborne Infections

Staying away from heavily polluted and populated areas will reduce the risk of inhaling airborne infections. Some examples of these infections are common cold, flu, chickenpox, mumps, measles, and many others.

Therefore, if you plan to exercise outside, make sure that you will breathe fresh air and not pollution. Some cities have small parks, but they may not be as healthy as you think during a busy time of the day. Try doing your exercise very early in the morning to avoid the pollution from vehicles.[348]

Day 281 – Breathing Fresh Air May Alleviate Asthma

It has been observed that the need for asthma medications is significantly decreased when there is good ventilation at home. Breathing fresh cold air can help alleviate asthma.

Dust mites, which thrive in humid environments, are one of the chief causes of asthma. Air conditioners can help because they remove heat and moisture from the air, reducing issues like dust mites.[349; 350]

Day 282 – Breathing Fresh Air May Alleviate Fatigue

Lack of oxygen can make us feel tired easily and discourage us from engaging in physical activities. Being physically inactive can lower our stamina in the long run. Exercising allows your blood to flow better all over your body, so it can also allow the oxygen to travel to the muscles and alleviate fatigue.

Go outside, breathe some fresh air, and do some stretching.[351]

Day 283 – Breathing Fresh Air May Increase Memory Capacity

The brain needs constant supply of oxygen. Without oxygen, we would be lifeless in minutes! Studying in a park or in your home garden may not be a bad idea. There could be visual and auditory distractions in a park, but your brain would benefit from the abundant supply of fresh air.[352]

Day 284 – Breathing Fresh Air May Boost Concentration

If you need to boost your concentration, make sure you are breathing enough oxygen and not air pollution. Breathing fresh air can give us a sharper mind and better overall cognitive function. Stressed at work? Instead of having a cigarette break (which can be very bad for your body), take a walk in a nearby park. Appreciate what nature can give you.[353]

Day 285 – Breathing Fresh Air Can Detoxify Your Body

The liver naturally detoxifies the body, but it heavily relies on oxygen to function properly. Lack of oxygen supply could result in liver damage. Breathing fresh air with plenty of oxygen could assist the liver in functioning properly and help detoxify your body.

You may have used detox supplements in the past. I'm not against anything that could help our bodies be healthier, but they could be quite expensive. In fact, you don't need any of those. There are plenty of things you can do naturally without breaking your wallet, like eating healthy foods, getting enough sleep, and being physically active.[354]

Day 286 – Breathing Fresh Air Can Reduce Stress

Research shows that oxygen contributes to the release of serotonin in the body, the hormone that is responsible for stabilizing our mood. If you are stressed out due to any variety of reasons, help your body relax by breathing fresh air. Go to someplace quiet and full of trees and plants.[355]

Day 287 – Breathing Fresh Air May Alleviate Anxiety

Anxiety causes shortness of breath, or what we call hyperventilation. If you are having an anxiety attack, it can help greatly if you focus on your breathing and then go to a place where you can breathe fresh air. If you don't have immediate access to fresh air, breathe slowly into a paper bag, or just cup your hands and breathe slowly into them.[356]

Day 288 – Breathing Fresh Air May Promote Better Sleep

Breathing less oxygen during sleep can cause serious health problems. This happens to people with obstructive sleep apnea who snore loudly and still feel exhausted even after a complete sleep. However, it could also happen to healthy people sleeping in a place without ample supply of fresh air and oxygen.

If you use air-conditioners while you sleep, make sure to have them cleaned regularly. Dirty filters can worsen asthma and may cause a lung infection, even if you are completely healthy. If you have a choice to open your windows and use fans for ventilation instead, that would be better.[357]

Day 289 – Breathing Fresh Air Can Prevent Lactic Acid Build-Up

Exercising produces lactic acid in the muscles. If it builds up, it can cause muscle soreness and cramps. Breathing fresh air with plenty of oxygen could break down the lactic acid to become carbon dioxide and water. That's why it's still best to exercise in a park filled with trees rather than in an air-conditioned gym.[358]

Day 290 – Breathing Fresh Air Can Prevent Color Changes in Your Vision

Studies show that inhaling less oxygen can affect the colors that the eyes can see. This is more evident in people who live in or travel to high-altitude places such as mountains because the higher you go up, the thinner the air gets.[359]

Day 291 – Breathing Fresh Air Can Make Exercise More Tolerable

During exercise or any strenuous activities, the body uses more oxygen. To aid that oxygen requirement, breathing also increases. It can be more beneficial to exercise in areas with many trees and less air pollution to help make exercise more tolerable and enjoyable.[360]

Day 292 – Breathing Fresh Air Can Help You Recover from Shortness of Breath

In a healthy person, shortness of breath can be experienced through doing a strenuous physical activity or just being in a high altitude. It's completely normal unless you have a disease such as pneumonia or asthma.

Breathing fresh air without any pollutants can help you recover from shortness of breath quicker. If it happens to persist and becomes unusually uncomfortable, go to the nearest hospital or clinic for immediate treatment and to determine its cause.[361]

Day 293 – Breathing Fresh Air Can Prolong Life by Reducing Heart Strain

Studies show that regularly breathing fresh air lowers the risk of heart attacks and relaxes the body overall, significantly reducing heart strain.

If you have an existing heart condition, it may greatly benefit your health if you regularly walk in parks. That's right, for this benefit, you don't just sit and breathe fresh air. You also need to walk, which is a basic form of exercise. See Chapter 6 to learn the benefits of walking![362]

Day 294 – Breathing Fresh Air May Prevent Inflammation

Low oxygen levels are directly linked to inflammation. If you already have inflammation, may it be skin or gut inflammation, it can be aggravated by lack of oxygen, so make sure you are breathing enough fresh air.

However, if you have severe inflammation, make sure to strictly follow your doctor's advice and prescriptions.[363]

Day 295 – Breathing Fresh Air May Help Treat Cough

Cough worsens in cold and dry environments. If you have a cough, going outside to get some sunshine and fresh air could help alleviate cough. If you have a dry cough, limit the use of air-conditioners because they remove humidity in the air.[364]

Day 296 – Breathing Fresh Air May Prevent Bone Mass Loss

Did you know that low oxygen levels are directly linked to bone mass loss? The oxygen we breathe goes to the blood, and 10% of the blood pumped by the heart is received by the bones. Reduced supply of oxygen to the bones through the blood could result in bone loss.

Exercising promotes stronger muscles and bones. Doing it in a place with fresh air will make them even stronger.[365]

Day 297 – Breathing Fresh Air May Prevent Lung Cancer

Lung cancer is the number one killer cancer in the US and the leading cause is cigarette smoking. However, outdoor air pollution can cause lung cancer as well. The youngest lung cancer patient in China as of this writing is an 8-year-old girl who developed the disease through air pollution.

If you are going to a heavily polluted environment, wearing certain face masks could help filter out some of the air pollutants. Take every opportunity to breathe fresh air to avoid lung cancer.[366]

Day 298 – Breathing Fresh Air May Prevent Hypoxemia

Breathing fresh air can prevent hypoxemia, or lack of oxygen in the blood. Hypoxemia can cause headaches and shortness of breath. When not treated, it can cause more serious conditions such as impaired brain and heart functions.[367]

Day 299 – Breathing Fresh Air May Help Metabolize Fat and Carbohydrates

Fats and carbohydrates, which are main energy sources, can be metabolized better by breathing fresh air. Just had a bountiful meal? Instead of sitting on the couch and watching TV, take a stroll and breathe fresh air. Walking after eating can help with your digestion, but do not brisk-walk or it could upset your stomach.[368]

Day 300 – Breathing Fresh Air May Help Patients with Pneumonia

An abundant supply of oxygen and fresh air can be extremely necessary for patients with pneumonia. Depending on the severity, you may even need to go to a hospital to use a breathing machine or ventilator.

Stay away from any smoke and polluted air if you have pneumonia. Pneumonia is usually caused by inhaled viruses and bacteria, so you should find a good place that is away from air pollution to recover.[369]

Key Takeaways

I know that most of us do not have much of a choice over the kind of environment where we live. Good places are not just expensive, they are also limited. You might not get the place you want even if you have the money.

If you live in a crowded city, chances are that the quality of air is way poorer as it is highly urbanized. There are fewer trees and more cars. More pollution means poorer air quality, and you could be more susceptible to lung infections. In this case, you might want to buy indoor plants to help freshen up the air even just a little bit. They are not expensive and easy to take care of, so it's a very good deal.

Go to parks once in a while to breathe fresh air. Take the opportunity to exercise and do some grounding, which we discussed in Chapter 5.

Also, avoid inhaling secondhand smoke, and of course, you should not smoke. I know it can be very difficult for some to quit. If you can't stop, you can seek help from a medical professional to guide you. Smoking is killing thousands of people around the world. In the US alone, almost half a million people die each year because of cigarette smoking. Sadly, more than 41,000 of those die because of secondhand smoke. Please, if you can't stop smoking, do not let others inhale your smoke. Don't infect those who do their best to stay healthy.

Month 11 – Meditate

Meditation is a practice wherein a person uses a method or technique to increase focus and mindfulness to achieve a clear mind and a stable emotional state. It is an ancient tradition that goes back thousands of years. In the Bible, the word meditate is first mentioned in the book of Genesis, and it is said to mean "to be absorbed in thought" or "to be thoughtful".

Meditation is used most commonly by people who are affiliated with religious organizations. However, one can meditate without being spiritual. It can be used for literally anything, such as sports, business, and health. For example, when you are stressed out and you're all over the place, you might want to sit down and compose yourself.

There are many different ways to meditate. What works for you may not be effective for others, but the objective is the same.

This chapter will not dissect the different methods of meditation. We will focus on its benefits to help you understand why it is important and why you should start doing it if you aren't already.

Day 301 – Meditation Can Help You Gain a New Perspective in Stressful Situations

Being in a stressful situation can give you a mental block, especially if you are caught by surprise. Focusing your mind on how to solve the problem and throwing away those extra thoughts could help you think of a solution sooner.

For example, your boss told you that you made a big mistake in your task, and it needs to be fixed as soon as possible. Instead of panicking, clear your mind for a moment and then gather your thoughts. If it helps, list down the things you should do so you have a visual aid that you can follow while you are fixing the problem.

Meditating while taking a walk can help, too. See how all of your new healthy habits are starting to come together?[370]

Day 302 – Meditation Can Help You Manage Stress Better

Some people encounter stress every day and too much stress can lead to various health problems.

Your overall health, including your mental health, should always be a priority. Even if you have a very tight schedule, make some time to do meditation at least once a day for 15 minutes or so. Clearing your mind can ease your stress and may help you do your job better.[371]

Day 303 – Meditation Can Help You Increase Self-Awareness

There are two types of self-awareness: public and private. If you are self-aware publicly, it means you are aware of how people look at you or how you appear to others. On the other hand, private awareness is becoming aware of what you feel personally and understanding your emotions.

Meditation can bring self-awareness as you let go of the negative or harmful thoughts and focus on what's important. It can be beneficial not only to you but to others as well. Give yourself a few minutes to meditate on the different emotions you are experiencing to learn something about yourself today.[372]

Day 304 – Meditation Can Help You Be Mindful of the Present

Sometimes, we think so much of the future that we ignore what's happening at the present time. While it is important to prepare and think for the future, we must also be mindful of the present, because that's when we can act and do something. Meditation can be used to help us redirect our focus to the present.

Pause for a moment and think of what you can do at the present. Think of the ways you utilize your time and how you are productive.[373]

Day 305 – Meditation Can Help You Manage Negative Emotions

Stressful situations can lead to many negative emotions. When we are engulfed with negative emotions, we could become unproductive because we focus our energy on what's negative and unhelpful.

Meditation may allow you to compose yourself so that you can address those negative emotions more effectively. Remember, you do not totally suppress your emotions. Let it out if that would make you more relieved, but control how you let it out.[374]

Day 306 – Meditation Can Help You Be More Imaginative and Creative

When meditating, you can free up your brain of the less useful thoughts and focus on what you really want to think. It can be a way to train yourself to get rid of the "noise" that stops your creative process.

For example, you are a designer in an advertising company, and you what to come up with new designs that could sell well. Meditation could allow you to boost your imagination and even remember past experiences that could help at the present.[375; 376]

Day 307 – Meditation Can Help You Increase Patience and Tolerance

Meditating can help you endure the things that test your patience. For example, if you have an annoying neighbor (who is noisy at night, for example), instead of losing your composure and yelling at them, you could pause for a moment and think of what you can say peacefully. Minimize the damage in your relationship with them as their neighbor and meditate on helpful solutions.

Many people get into fights because of misunderstandings. Let meditation help you avoid engaging in unnecessary quarrels and instead build stronger, peaceful relationships.[377]

Day 308 – Meditation May Help Reduce Anxiety

While you may need professional help with your anxiety, meditation could alleviate what you feel. We may become anxious because of various problems in life. This could include relationships, finances, family, and many others.

Try going someplace where you can be comfortable, do some breathing exercises, and contemplate on your problems one by one. Carefully address each problem while keeping a calm mind.[378]

Day 309 – Meditation May Help Alleviate Asthma

Asthma is the inflammation of the airways that makes it hard to breathe. If you're stressed, your body can release chemicals that can aggravate or cause inflammation, so your asthma can be affected as well.

Along with medications you may be prescribed (which you should take as directed), meditation can alleviate stress by practicing mindfulness and inducing relaxation. Instead of overthinking, clear your mind for a moment and concentrate on the present time. Do breathing exercises along with it.[379]

Day 310 – Meditation May Help Fight Cancer

Fighting cancer is probably one of the hardest things we may experience. The treatment is expensive and there is no guarantee of full recovery, especially in the latter stages. This condition could bring a great deal of stress to a person. Chemotherapy could even cause emotional instability.

Meditation is very much recommended to cancer patients to alleviate stress and to keep a positive mind. If you are a cancer patient, it could help significantly if you could find a meditation expert to carefully guide you throughout your recovery.[380]

Day 311 – Meditation May Help Alleviate Chronic Pain

Did you know that meditation can help with pain? A study showed that those who attended meditation programs reported significantly less pain than those who did not do any meditation.

Long-term meditation practice may positively affect the cortical thickness of parts of the brain involved in pain processing. Cortical thinning, on the other hand, is associated with brain diseases such as dementia and Parkinson's disease.

Take some time to meditate. It can be very beneficial for your mental health.[381]

Day 312 – Meditation May Help Fight Depression

Not all people can afford a therapist to help them treat their depression. Meditation is a free and relatively easy method which can aid in reducing the severity of depression.

Meditation allows you to be self-aware physically and mentally. It can help you control your negative thoughts by focusing your attention on other things such as self-compassion.

However, the positive effects of meditation do not happen overnight. It takes time and practice. You must make an effort, spend time with yourself, and love yourself.[382]

Day 313 – Meditation May Help Fight Heart Disease

Meditation may promote heart health by lowering the blood pressure and helping to fight addictions that could be harmful to the heart, such as smoking. Also, long-term stress is a risk for heart disease. Regular meditation could help manage stress, thus potentially preventing you from developing heart problems.[383]

Day 314 – Meditation May Help Stabilize Blood Pressure

Meditation may help lower blood pressure by inducing relaxation. When you are relaxed, your blood vessels widen, and blood pressure is lowered as a result.

Anger could raise your blood pressure, so learning the techniques of meditation can help you be in control of your emotions and thoughts.[384]

Day 315 – Meditation May Help Treat Irritable Bowel Syndrome

Studies show that meditation could help people with irritable bowel syndrome (IBS) by lowering their stress levels and reducing anxiety associated with IBS. While meditation does not cure IBS, it could reduce the severity of the disease. It can be important to be calm and practice positive thinking when recovering from a disease.[385]

Day 316 – Meditation May Promote Better Sleep

Sleep disorders are often caused by stress and anxiety. Maybe you cannot sleep because there are lots of things going on in your mind that you want to resolve but you can't at the moment. If this is the reason why you cannot sleep, meditation can greatly help you.

Start by making your place of sleep comfortable. Turn off the lights (or use dim lights if you are not comfortable with total darkness). Remove any distractions like sources of noise if possible. Lie on your back and do breathing exercises while relaxing your whole body. Let go of any thoughts, whether they are positive or negative. Focus on your breathing. It may be more effective if you do all of these while your eyes are closed. Now that you are relaxed, it may be easier for you to sleep.[386]

Day 317 – Meditation May Reduce Tension Headaches

A study was done involving the use of rajyoga meditation for patients experiencing chronic tension-type headaches. One group was taught and made to meditate on top of medical treatment involving analgesics and muscle relaxants, while another group just received the analgesics and muscle relaxants. Results show that headache relief, as calculated by headache index, was 99% in the meditation group as compared to 51% in the medical treatment-only group. This means that meditation was highly effective in reducing headache.[387]

Day 318 – Meditation Can Help You Relax

Meditation can help you relax deeply by regulating your thoughts and focusing on the present moment. Remembering a good experience may also help during meditation. It can be something spiritual or a past memory that makes you more motivated. Listening to relaxing music at low volume while meditating may also help.[388]

Day 319 – Meditation Can Help You Make Better Judgments

Meditation allows you to spend time with yourself. It is a solitary moment that you can use to reflect on things while maintaining relaxation.

If you are about to make a big decision and you are still unsure of what to do, meditate for a while and find your inner peace. Whatever conforms with your inner peace, that is most probably the correct decision.

Always remember not to rush things, especially if you have the time to ponder.[389]

Day 320 – Meditation May Help You Focus

One of the requirements of meditation is focusing on the present moment. Regular meditation practice can help you improve your focus when needed.

For example, a problem arises at work that you need to resolve immediately. If you have practiced meditation for some time, it could be easier for you to focus on the problem and not panic.[390]

Day 321 – Meditation May Help You Accept Reality

Part of meditation is being mindful of what you currently feel physically and emotionally. It can allow you to let go of thoughts about things that are not really going to happen. We may have regrets that constantly haunt us. Meditation can greatly help us overcome regrets of things we cannot change and accept what is real in the present.[391; 392]

Day 322 – Meditation May Help Alleviate Fibromyalgia

Patients diagnosed with fibromyalgia can greatly benefit from mindfulness meditation. Studies show that meditation helps in attenuating pain, thus reducing the severity of the disease. Meditation that focuses on acceptance, non-attachment, and social engagement, in addition to nonjudgmental awareness, appears to be most effective in improving fibromyalgia-related outcomes.[393]

Day 323 – Meditation May Help Treat Post-Traumatic Stress Disorder (PTSD)

Studies have shown that meditation as well as yoga can help in the treatment of PTSD among adults through benefits such as reducing stress, inducing relaxation, non-judgmental observation of thoughts and feelings, and controlling intrusive memories. If you are experiencing PTSD, talk to your doctor about how to include meditation in your treatment plan.[394]

Day 324 – Meditation May Increase Memory

Are you becoming forgetful? Studies have shown that daily meditation decreases negative mood and enhances attention, working memory, and recognition memory.

Some people are so busy that they do not have their alone time anymore. Our mental health is as important as our physical health. Take some time to breathe, ponder on things, and relax. If you feel the need to relax because you are just drowned with so many things, perhaps take several days off. Take care of yourself.[395]

Day 325 – Meditation May Prevent Development of Alzheimer's Disease

A study was done specifically for the Kirtan Kriya meditation. The results show that 12-minute daily Kirtan Kriya meditation improves the memory of people with cognitive decline and with mild cognitive impairment, which are risks of developing Alzheimer's disease.

Meditation can be a vital piece of our daily lives. Healthy diet and regular exercise are important, but meditation is of the same importance. Our mental health is just as important as our physical health. Take a few minutes to relax, breathe, and meditate today.[396]

Day 326 – Meditation May Offset Age-Related Cognitive Decline

Studies have shown that meditation can offset age-related cognitive decline by its positive effects on attention, memory, executive function, processing speed, and general cognition.

As we grow old, our cognitive power becomes weaker, as well as our bodies, but we should not let old age get the best of us! Meditation can help stimulate brain activity, so we should do it regularly to prevent cognitive decline.[397]

Day 327 – Meditation May Help Reduce Psychological Distress for Dementia Caregivers

Dementia caregivers are known to have an increased risk of adverse mental health sequalae. Studies have shown that meditation could help dementia caregivers in alleviating their depression, burden, and stress.

If you are taking care of a family member who has dementia, meditation can help you cope with the situation. Take care of yourself as well.[398]

Day 328 – Meditation May Generate Kindness

If you want to do good things from the heart, meditation can
help you to be kinder to others. Kindness involves understanding
other people's needs and problems. If you focus on other people
rather than yourself, it will manifest in your actions. Meditation
can only generate genuine kindness if you have a good heart.
Remember, good actions only become good if the intentions are
pure.[399]

Day 329 – Meditation May Boost Empathy

Sometimes, we become so self-absorbed that we forget to listen to others. If you want to understand a person, meditation can help you empathize more as you focus on the other person's needs above yours. Meditation can allow you to reflect on things and be aware of everything that you do.

If you notice that the people around you are becoming distant, maybe something is off with your perspective. The sooner you determine what's wrong, the sooner you can fix your relationships with them. While your happiness is important, if you focus too much on your own happiness, the tendency is that you lose empathy. Take some time to meditate and think of your recent behaviors. How would you feel on the other side of the interaction?[400]

Day 330 – Meditation May Help Fight Addictions

There aren't many people who can leave their addictions cold turkey because it can be extremely difficult to do. Long-time smokers, for example, could find it very difficult to quit smoking because they are attached to the smell of cigarettes and the sensation that it brings to the body.

Meditation could assist you in leaving your addiction. For example, understanding the bad effects of smoking can stir up the fear of dying. Focusing on what's more important – which is your life and health – can help you let go of things that are harmful to you.[401]

Key Takeaways

I hope you have learned something from this chapter. You may not have expected meditation to be a part of a health book, but it has genuine importance to our mental health. In fact, you may have been already doing meditation without realizing.

If you are not yet aware of meditation techniques, there are lots of materials and videos on the internet. You can also buy books from your local bookstore or from Amazon. If you can find a meditation expert who can teach you personally, all the better! I encourage you to explore meditation because it can help you to be more open and more rational.

At the end of the day, it is up to you to determine the focus of your meditations. Meditation just allows you to channel your energy to what's more important for you. It does not always point you in the right direction. Always ask yourself what your motivation is. Does it conform with moral standards? Does it agree with your conscience, perhaps? Meditation can only be truly beneficial if you meditate on things that are morally upright, otherwise it could even be harmful.

Month 12 – Practice a Daily Affirmation

Congratulations! You have reached the final chapter! We have already discussed so much information about the health benefits of different foods, supplements, and practices. In this chapter, we will finally discuss affirming oneself.

Affirmations are phrases or mantras which state things about oneself that may or may not be true. For example, if you tell yourself, "I am an adorable person," two things could happen: (1) you blindly believe that you are an adorable person and you become annoying to others, or (2) you become constantly self-aware of your actions with the goal of improving yourself to be adorable.

In the previous chapter, we discussed how our true intentions ultimately guide us in life. Whatever we do, including affirmations, will be guided in a direction based on our motivations. In the US TV show *The Good Place*, one of the main characters, Tahani, raised millions of dollars for charity, but she didn't really care about the poor. She just wanted to get her parents' approval. While giving to the poor is good, it will not count as a "good" act if the motivation is corrupt.

The reason why I'm saying this is because you may misunderstand the goal of this chapter. Self-affirmation can only be healthy and helpful if you do it right. Just like body exercises, you must know how to execute them properly to avoid injuries.

Before you continue, you must know that there are studies showing that present tense positive affirmations (e.g., "I am" statements) are only effective for people who have high self-esteem and can be detrimental to those who have low self-esteem. However, using future tense positive affirmations (e.g., "I will" statements) is found to be effective for people who have low self-esteem. The examples mentioned in this chapter use "I am," but you can change the phrases to the future tense "I will" if you feel you have lower self-esteem as you complete these daily affirmations.

Day 331 – Affirmations Can Help You Stay Motivated

There are a lot of things that can bring your motivation down. Sometimes, just a simple side comment from someone can affect your mood for the entire day.

Do a self-affirmation like this one: In the morning before going to work, try telling yourself, *"I am very happy with what I'm doing and I'm making a positive impact on other people."*

Telling yourself that you're happy may give you a mood boost. However, if you are not actually happy because of valid reasons like having a toxic workplace, positive affirmations may not help at all. Remember that daily affirmations are not lying to yourself. It is reminding yourself of what's real. However, it could still positively affect your mood and make the best out of bad situations.[402]

Day 332 – Affirmations Can Help You Feel Secure

If you do not feel secure, it could mean you are anxious about something. We all have those moments when we are very vulnerable and we tend to seek comfort, but there is not always someone who could comfort us and make us feel secure.

Whenever you feel vulnerable, try telling yourself something like, *"I am strong and independent. I can survive without constant support from other people."*

Sometimes, we just forget to believe in our capabilities. If you keep thinking you are weak, you will not be able to move forward because that's your mindset. Changing your mindset can also change your actions.[403]

Day 333 – Affirmations May Help You Keep a Rational Mind

Sometimes, when we are overwhelmed by emotions or desires, we tend to be illogical and make bad decisions.

Try telling yourself, *"I am keeping an open mind no matter what happens."*

Telling yourself this can help you keep your cool. If we keep a rational mind, we can dodge huge mistakes. I'm not saying that we should always contain our emotions, don't get me wrong. Sometimes, letting go of our emotions is the better option. You can be angry, but remember to keep it at bay. Meaning, don't do something stupid and reckless. Express your emotions in an appropriate manner instead.[404]

Day 334 – Affirmations Can Encourage You to Do the Right Thing

We all have our weaknesses, and sometimes doing the right thing is the hardest thing to do. On the other hand, if we keep doing what's morally unacceptable, it could eventually corrupt our moral standards.

Have you encountered people who just seem twisted, like the ones who believe that beating their partners is acceptable? We do not want to end up like those people, so I encourage you to always remind yourself to do what is right.

Try telling yourself, *"I am always happy to help others."*[405]

Day 335 – Affirmations Can Boost Confidence

Those who are confident succeed in life, even if they don't have a lot of skill. Lack of self-confidence could stress you out, so you must begin working on it. For starters, you could try this self-affirmation to boost your confidence.

"I am always delighted to take every good opportunity."

Just think of all the opportunities that could be wasted because of lack of confidence. Affirm yourself today to potentially avoid missing out tomorrow.[406]

Day 336 – Affirmations May Allow You to Help Others Without Expecting in Return

It is normal to expect something in return when you help, but it is much better if you help without expecting anything in return. If you always expect favors to be returned to you, you may be disappointed. Not all people return a favor or offer anything as a thank you, and that's reality.

Try telling yourself, *"I am always happy to help, even if they do not return the favor."*

It's called being selfless. It could also give you a sense of self-fulfillment that can affect your overall mood positively. Start by doing something small.[407]

Day 337 – Affirmations Could Bring Awareness of Your Abilities

Sometimes, we are not aware of our own abilities because we fail to discover them or are reluctant to do so.

Try telling yourself, *"I am not afraid to try new things, or else I will be stagnant and miss many good opportunities."*

Not knowing your abilities or capabilities may leave you stuck in a place without growth. Who knows? Maybe you have a talent in hosting or in sales. Affirming yourself could help you find the willingness to try new things.[408]

Day 338 – Affirmations Can Help You Recognize What Makes You Proud

We occasionally do not recognize our small achievements because we think they are insignificant. However, these small achievements can help define our capabilities, and we should be proud of them.

Try telling yourself, *"I am proud of the way I organized my things in my apartment."*

Yes, it feels good if other people recognize your accomplishments, but you should also recognize them yourself. What you should avoid is bragging about them to other people no matter how subtle. You do not seek or ask for affirmation, you affirm yourself.[409]

Day 339 – Affirmations Could Allow You to Grow and Learn

Excuses are always there to hinder us from growing. Overcome those excuses, stand up, and do what you need to do. Successful people did not become successful overnight. They took risks and made serious efforts on things that they wanted to achieve. If we are not motivated, it is highly unlikely for us to grow and learn new things.

Try telling yourself something like, *"I have no excuses and I am more than happy to challenge myself to learn new things."*[410]

Day 340 – Affirmations May Allow You to Be the Person You Want to Be

Sometimes, we are shy or hesitant to pursue our passion because we lack faith in ourselves and listen to what other people say instead. If you always worry about what other people think, you can bring a lot of stress on yourself. Opinions of other people will never end.

Try telling yourself something like, *"I am who I am, and I do not care what other people say as long as I'm not doing anything wrong."*

As long as you're not doing anything wrong, be yourself, but remember to always be mindful, because sometimes, what we think is right may be socially or morally unacceptable.[411]

Day 341 – Affirmations May Allow You to Trust Your Gut While Being Rational

We all have our "gut feeling." It's like something is telling us what to do, or not to do, or else something bad will happen. Sometimes, we do not follow our guts because we are afraid of the outcome.

Try telling yourself something like, *"I am mature and wise enough to trust my gut."*

Our gut feeling is usually correct because our past experiences and cumulative knowledge guide us in the current situation. If you're still unsure of what to do, ask other people. In my experience, I always learn something from good conversations with others, so it can be wise to talk to other people.[412]

Day 342 – Affirmations May Allow You to Accept Your Emotions

What we feel is valid and we should not stop ourselves from feeling our emotions. Sometimes, we are just afraid to face reality, so we convey a different emotion, but we are fooling ourselves if we do that.

Tell yourself something like, *"I am happy to express my own emotions and it liberates me."*

We are free to express our emotions, but we should know how to control them as well. For example, there are people with anger management issues who cannot control their anger. There are also people who cry a lot because they cannot control their sadness. If you think you are experiencing an unnatural burst of emotions, you could consult a medical professional.[413]

Day 343 – Affirmations May Help You Give Yourself the Care and Attention You Deserve

There are people who are selfless and are always attending to the needs of other people. If you are this kind of person, I commend you, but if you are depriving yourself of care for too long, it could burn you out.

Tell yourself something like, *"I am important, and I care for myself and my needs."*

Caring for yourself does not mean that you are being selfish. It is keeping the balance between caring for others and caring for yourself. Feel free to treat and reward yourself how and when it is appropriate.[414]

Day 344 – Affirmations May Help You Reach Your Goals

Sometimes, we inhibit ourselves from reaching our goals because we are afraid of the outcome, or maybe we overthink the process of reaching them.

Try telling yourself something like this: *"I am completely decided with my goals, and I am going to reach them no matter what."*

Maybe not all of our goals will materialize, but it's better to try than to not start at all. We only live once and we can only do so much in our lifetime, so don't just sit there. Get out there and start achieving![415]

Day 345 – Affirmations May Help You Share What You Can Do

There are people who are too shy to showcase their talents and abilities. Your talents and abilities can make a positive impact on others, perhaps even the world.

Try telling yourself something like this: *"I am happy to share what I know to help others."*

Sharing what you can do and bragging about what you can do are two different things. Always be humble no matter what.[416]

Day 346 – Affirmations Can Help You Keep a Clear Mind

Indecisiveness is a blocker to our goals. Yes, there are times that we reach a slump, but it should be temporary. Anxiety also messes with our decision-making, so we should work on that first if we are experiencing it.

Tell yourself something like, *"I am sure of what I want to do, and I know that it is the right thing."*

If you have already thought of something many times over and you reach the same conclusion, then go for it. Self-affirmation may help with confusion as it allows you to clear your mind of other thoughts which could be harmful.[417]

Day 347 – Affirmations May Provide Constant Inspiration

Losing inspiration may lead to depression, which we don't want to happen. We must always find something that fuels our inspiration. It could be another person or a goal, whatever works for you. If you are a parent, your inspiration could be your children. It can be important to always be inspired because it can push us to move forward and accomplish things.

Tell yourself something like, *"I am good at what I do, and I will continue to improve one step at a time."*[418]

Day 348 – Affirmations Can Boost Your Creativity and Innovativeness

All of us can be creative, but sometimes we are just not inspired enough to think outside the box.

Try telling yourself something like, *"I am good enough to think of new ideas."*

If you think you are not good enough, ideas will not come to your mind. Even the brightest people can't think straight if they are depressed or unmotivated. It's not just our IQ. What drives us is also important. If you have a sports car but it doesn't have gas, it wouldn't run at all. The same can be said for us if we have lost our inspiration.[419]

Day 349 – Affirmations Can Help You Channel Your Energy to the Most Important Things

Sometimes we focus our energy on the most trivial of things, like spending too much time browsing the web. We have limited energy to spend throughout the day. We must know how to spend it wisely.

Before going to work, try telling yourself something like, *"I am focusing my energy on my job today and will finish all my tasks."*

We can overwork when required, but it could bring us fatigue and all sorts of discomfort. Be sure to prioritize your health and use affirmations to remind you to use your time wisely.[420]

Day 350 – Affirmations May Allow You to Trust Yourself in Making Right Decisions

Sometimes, we lose trust in ourselves when we make a series of bad decisions. If you feel you are lost and cannot trust yourself, seek advice from people you trust. If you don't have anyone to talk to at the moment, think of the right decisions you've made in the past to remind you that you are capable.

Try telling yourself something like, *"I am sufficient and capable, and I know I can make the right decisions."*[421]

Day 351 – Affirmations Can Allow You to Know Your True Self

If you are a people-pleaser type of person, you may lose your own identity and personality because you always adjust yourself for others.

Tell yourself something like, *"I have my own identity, and I am happy with who I am."*

Of course, we must also improve and mature through time and be a better person every day. If you are having a hard time overcoming people-pleasing, try consulting a psychologist to help you out. They are experts in human behavior who may be able to help you care for yourself once and for all.[422]

Day 352 – Affirmations May Help with Gratitude

It is important to feel grateful of other people who have helped you. It will make you feel happy and inspired to help others as well. A simple "Thank you" is enough to convey our gratefulness to others. Sometimes we just forget to say it because we think the help that we received is trivial. While humble people do not seek out being thanked, it can make someone's day if you appreciate their efforts for you.

Tell yourself something like, *"I am grateful to all the people who have helped me no matter how small the act."*[423]

Day 353 – Affirmations Can Help You Learn Lessons Every Day

We can learn something from every day of our lives, even if it's something small. We must always be willing to learn no matter how wise and knowledgeable we think we are. Knowledge is virtually endless. Listen even to the people who you think know less than you. We have different experiences in life, so we can always learn something from each other.

Before you start your day, tell yourself something like, *"I always keep an open mind so I can always learn something."*[124]

Day 354 – Affirmations Can Help Us Find Inner Peace

Inner peace can be one of the most important things we should acquire in life. People with inner peace can be unlikely to have anxiety and depression because they always try to see the best in all situations.

Try to tell yourself something like, *"I am secure and settled, and I am sure that there is always a solution to every problem."*

Achieving inner peace is difficult to work on, but it is not impossible. One of the things we can do to achieve inner peace is not to harbor anger. I know it's difficult to forgive sometimes, but the truth is, it can benefit our health if we genuinely forgive.[425]

Day 355 – Affirmations Can Assist with Knowing That You Make a Difference in the World

You are just one of the billions of people in the world, but you are making a difference, even if people do not seem to notice it.

Tell yourself something like, *"I am significant, and I know I can make the world a better place even in my own little way."*

Even if you are just a lowly person with no social status whatsoever, you can make a difference by making other people happy, like by greeting them, "Good morning," or saying, "You look good today."[426]

Day 356 – Affirmations Can Help You Take Control of Your Life

Sometimes we forget that we control our own lives. Even if we are working 8-10 hours a day in a big corporation, we can still do a lot of things after work. We can also take time off from work and do what we want to do in our personal time.

Tell yourself something like, *"I am determined to pursue my dreams, and I am not afraid to move when needed."*

Your life is yours to control. Pursue your dreams as long as you are not doing anything wrong.[427]

Day 357 – Affirmations Can Help You Control Negative Thoughts

If you are too occupied with negative thoughts, you should do something about it, or else it could eat you up inside.

Tell yourself something like, *"I am optimistic that everything will be okay."*

Problems come and go, and the best way to solve them is to face them one by one. If you think you are too deep into having negative thoughts, talk to your family and friends. They may be able to help you out.[428]

Day 358 – Affirmations Can Help You Learn to Forgive

Forgiveness is part of our lives. You may choose not to forgive, but the truth is, it's not healthy mentally or physically.

Tell yourself something like, *"I am always ready to forgive, because at the end of the day, hatred does not do anything good."*

The easier you can forgive, the easier you can move on to the next chapter of your life. Remaining angry can just stress you out.[429]

Day 359 – Affirmations Can Help You Learn to Be Compassionate

Being compassionate is part of being human. Every day is not always a good day. Some are stricken with misfortune, and we must always be willing to extend help.

Tell yourself something like, *"I am a compassionate person, and I am willing to help others whenever I can."*

Helping others sincerely can be fulfilling. Moreover, if you are the one in need, you may not feel guilty asking for support because you also help others.[430]

Day 360 – Affirmations Can Help You Realize Your Potential

It is important to realize your potential because it can help you determine what you want to do with your life. There are people who discover their potential and abilities late in life because they were either lazy or hesitant when they were young. Time flies and we don't want to grow old full of regrets.

Tell yourself something like, *"I am always willing to try out new things to discover my potential."*[431]

Key Takeaways

Daily affirmations are shown to improve the lives of people who constantly use them. It's a mind conditioning technique wherein you focus your thoughts and energy to a particular belief or goal.

You may have done affirmations in the past, like telling yourself, *"I can do it!"* This may be the most common one. As we've discussed in this chapter, we can do all sorts of self-affirmations to help us in different aspects of life.

If we fail at something, it doesn't mean that we should stop. If all successful people stopped when they first encountered failure, they would not be where they are now. Most of the time, we just have to try and try, and daily affirmations can help you set your mind straight.

Closing

I have no idea if you've read ahead or waited until the end of the year to find these words. That means I have to speak to two different versions of you.

If you're reading ahead, it may mean that you're looking for the magic answer, the part of the book you can skip to and find the solution. The solution lies in small amounts of every page in this book. That may sound dismissive, but it's true. I've said it elsewhere in these pages – trust the process.

If you've just finished the year of actions, then let me be the first to congratulate you. Following a path like this one isn't easy. It takes dedication, and time, and a willingness to persist when it doesn't feel like your progress is as fast as you want it to be. But you did it, and you can now look back over the last year and see some real changes.

Well done!

What's next? I'd suggest you find some other simple actions you can add to your stack of habits. Once you get through a new action for a month, there's a good chance it gets much easier to keep going, which is why we constructed this book in this format.

No matter what you do, don't stop doing the new habits you've learned. Remember, today's results are based on yesterday's effort.

References

Month 1 – Drink One Large Glass of Water First Thing in the Morning

Introduction

1. https://www.usgs.gov/special-topic/water-science-school/science/water-you-water-and-human-body
2. https://www.washingtonpost.com/lifestyle/wellness/disregard-that-persistent-myth-you-can-drink-water-while-eating/2019/04/19/7f8f9b44-5ca6-11e9-a00e-050dc7b82693_story.html
3. https://www.healthline.com/health/food-nutrition/nine-types-of-drinking-water
4. https://en.wikipedia.org/wiki/Hunger_strike#Medical_view
5. https://www.businessinsider.com/how-many-days-can-you-survive-without-water-2014-5

Day 1

6. https://www.healthline.com/nutrition/drinking-water-in-the-morning

Day 2

7. https://www.ncbi.nlm.nih.gov/pmc/articles/PMC5615503/

Day 3

8. https://hub.jhu.edu/at-work/2020/01/15/focus-on-wellness-drinking-more-water/

Day 4

9. https://www.healthline.com/nutrition/drinking-water-helps-with-weight-loss

Day 5

10. https://www.ncbi.nlm.nih.gov/pmc/articles/PMC3445147/

Day 6

11. https://www.ncbi.nlm.nih.gov/pmc/articles/PMC3312700/
12. https://www.ncbi.nlm.nih.gov/pmc/articles/PMC5052503

Day 7

13. https://www.ncbi.nlm.nih.gov/books/NBK279392/

Day 8

14. https://www.cdc.gov/ncbddd/dvt/data.html
15. https://www.mayoclinic.org/symptoms/blood-clots/basics/causes/sym-20050850?p=1
16. https://academic.oup.com/qjmed/article/97/5/293/1555612

Day 9

17. https://www.ncbi.nlm.nih.gov/pmc/articles/PMC6629391/

Day 10

18. https://www.usgs.gov/special-topic/water-science-school/science/water-you-water-and-human-body
19. https://www.ncbi.nlm.nih.gov/pmc/articles/PMC4529263/

Day 11

20. https://www.ncbi.nlm.nih.gov/pmc/articles/PMC4325863/

Day 12

21. https://www.ncbi.nlm.nih.gov/pmc/articles/PMC6723555/

Day 13

22. https://www.ncbi.nlm.nih.gov/pmc/articles/PMC6723555/

Day 14

23. https://www.ncbi.nlm.nih.gov/pmc/articles/PMC6723555/

Day 15

24. https://www.ncbi.nlm.nih.gov/books/NBK507838/

Day 16

25. https://pubmed.ncbi.nlm.nih.gov/25950246/

Day 17

26. https://www.ncbi.nlm.nih.gov/pmc/articles/PMC6629391

Day 18

27. https://www.health.harvard.edu/diseases-and-conditions/lightheaded-top-5-reasons-you-might-feel-woozy

Day 19

28. https://www.ncbi.nlm.nih.gov/pmc/articles/PMC4606616/

Day 20

29. https://www.ncbi.nlm.nih.gov/pmc/articles/PMC5817324/

Day 21

30. https://www.ncbi.nlm.nih.gov/pmc/articles/PMC6282244/

Day 22

31. https://www.ncbi.nlm.nih.gov/pmc/articles/PMC2791660/

Day 23

32. https://pubmed.ncbi.nlm.nih.gov/359266/

Day 24

33. https://www.betterhealth.vic.gov.au/health/conditionsandtreatments/Tooth-decay

Day 25

34. https://pubmed.ncbi.nlm.nih.gov/25950246/

Day 26

35. https://www.healthline.com/health/thick-semen#other-causes

Day 27

36. https://solaramentalhealth.com/can-drinking-enough-water-help-my-depression-and-anxiety/

Day 28

37. https://www.healthline.com/nutrition/water-fasting

Day 29

38. https://www.ncbi.nlm.nih.gov/books/NBK235589/

Day 30

39. https://www.aquaidwatercoolers.co.uk/drinking-water-helps-you-breathe-easier#:~:text=Dehydration%20can%20cause%20that%20mucus,secretions%20that%20promote%20proper%20respiration

Month 2 – Start the Day with Fat

Day 31

40. https://www.sciencedaily.com/releases/2010/03/100330161751.htm

Day 32

41. https://pubmed.ncbi.nlm.nih.gov/9497173/

Day 33

42. https://pubmed.ncbi.nlm.nih.gov/9497173/
43. https://pubmed.ncbi.nlm.nih.gov/27457635/

Day 34

44. https://www.ncbi.nlm.nih.gov/pmc/articles/PMC4653532/

Day 35

45. https://pubmed.ncbi.nlm.nih.gov/16287956/

Day 36

46. https://pubmed.ncbi.nlm.nih.gov/8637339/

Day 37

47. https://pubmed.ncbi.nlm.nih.gov/11317662/

Day 38

48. https://www.psychologytoday.com/us/blog/your-brain-food/201205/dietary-fats-improve-brain-function

Day 39

49. https://www.healthline.com/nutrition/monounsaturated-fats#TOC_TITLE_HDR_7

Day 40

50. https://www.healthline.com/nutrition/17-health-benefits-of-omega-3#TOC_TITLE_HDR_2
51. https://www.ncbi.nlm.nih.gov/pmc/articles/PMC3976923/

Day 41

52. https://www.healthline.com/nutrition/17-health-benefits-of-omega-3#TOC_TITLE_HDR_3
53. https://pubmed.ncbi.nlm.nih.gov/15555528/

Day 42

54. https://www.healthline.com/nutrition/17-health-benefits-of-omega-3#TOC_TITLE_HDR_4
55. https://pubmed.ncbi.nlm.nih.gov/12509593/

Day 43

56. https://pubmed.ncbi.nlm.nih.gov/24934907/

Day 44

57. https://pubmed.ncbi.nlm.nih.gov/17493949/

Day 45

58. https://www.ncbi.nlm.nih.gov/pmc/articles/PMC3827145/

Day 46

59. https://pubmed.ncbi.nlm.nih.gov/7588501/

Day 47

60. https://pubmed.ncbi.nlm.nih.gov/24605819/

Day 48

61. https://www.ncbi.nlm.nih.gov/pmc/articles/PMC3435270/

Day 49

62. https://www.ncbi.nlm.nih.gov/pmc/articles/PMC4109685/

Day 50

63. https://www.ncbi.nlm.nih.gov/pmc/articles/PMC6413158/

Day 51

64. https://pubmed.ncbi.nlm.nih.gov/17384344/

Day 52

65. https://www.ncbi.nlm.nih.gov/pmc/articles/PMC3607650/

Day 53

    66. https://www.ncbi.nlm.nih.gov/pmc/articles/PMC3720090/

Day 54

    67. https://pubmed.ncbi.nlm.nih.gov/26263244/

Day 55

    68. https://pubmed.ncbi.nlm.nih.gov/11356585/

Day 56

    69. https://pubmed.ncbi.nlm.nih.gov/10232294/

Day 57

    70. https://pubmed.ncbi.nlm.nih.gov/2893189/

Day 58

    71. https://pubmed.ncbi.nlm.nih.gov/22023985/

Day 59

    72. https://pubmed.ncbi.nlm.nih.gov/17413117/

Day 60

    73. https://pubmed.ncbi.nlm.nih.gov/20980487/

Month 3 – The Beauty of Good Carbs

Day 61

74. https://pubmed.ncbi.nlm.nih.gov/21475137/

Day 62

75. https://www.healthline.com/nutrition/carbohydrate-functions#TOC_TITLE_HDR_2

Day 63

76. https://www.healthline.com/nutrition/carbohydrate-functions#TOC_TITLE_HDR_3

Day 64

77. https://www.healthline.com/nutrition/carbohydrate-functions#TOC_TITLE_HDR_4
78. https://inbodyusa.com/blogs/inbodyblog/why-you-need-carbs-to-build-muscle/#:~:text=Carbs%20are%20important%20for%20muscle,loss%20and%20help%20repair%20muscles

Day 65

79. https://pubmed.ncbi.nlm.nih.gov/21332763/

Day 66

80. https://www.healthline.com/nutrition/carbohydrate-functions#TOC_TITLE_HDR_5

Day 67

81. https://pubmed.ncbi.nlm.nih.gov/18039988/

Day 68

82. https://pubmed.ncbi.nlm.nih.gov/23422921/

Day 69

83. https://www.ncbi.nlm.nih.gov/pmc/articles/PMC4224210/
84. https://watermark.silverchair.com/nutritionreviews60-0155.pdf

Day 70

85. https://www.ncbi.nlm.nih.gov/pmc/articles/PMC4224210/
86. https://pubmed.ncbi.nlm.nih.gov/21332763/

Day 71

87. https://www.ncbi.nlm.nih.gov/pmc/articles/PMC4224210/
88. https://www.deccanchronicle.com/lifestyle/health-and-wellbeing/230417/why-carbohydrates-are-very-important-for-the-brain.html

Day 72

89. https://www.ncbi.nlm.nih.gov/pmc/articles/PMC4588743/

Day 73

90. https://www.ncbi.nlm.nih.gov/pmc/articles/PMC5348370/

Day 74

91. https://pubmed.ncbi.nlm.nih.gov/23539529/

Day 75

92. https://www.mayoclinic.org/healthy-lifestyle/nutrition-and-healthy-eating/in-depth/fiber/art-20043983
93. https://pubmed.ncbi.nlm.nih.gov/9925120/

Day 76

94. https://www.mayoclinic.org/healthy-lifestyle/nutrition-and-healthy-eating/in-depth/fiber/art-20043983
95. https://pubmed.ncbi.nlm.nih.gov/16407729

Day 77

96. https://pubmed.ncbi.nlm.nih.gov/24478050/

Day 78

97. https://pubmed.ncbi.nlm.nih.gov/25559238/

Day 79

98. https://www.health.com/food/18-health-benefits-of-whole-grains?slide=f74f25d4-e9a9-4908-ba0b-51ae21d18d3f#f74f25d4-e9a9-4908-ba0b-51ae21d18d3f

Day 80

99. https://www.health.com/food/18-health-benefits-of-whole-grains?slide=073d3157-5c50-489a-837e-3b6358d2039b#073d3157-5c50-489a-837e-3b6358d2039b

Day 81

    100. https://www.health.com/food/18-health-benefits-of-whole-grains?slide=d0f84476-b8ba-4379-9706-5d9b99cd8557#d0f84476-b8ba-4379-9706-5d9b99cd8557

Day 82

    101. https://www.health.com/food/18-health-benefits-of-whole-grains?slide=4f2a9ce9-8263-45d0-aa98-deda5cffe3e9#4f2a9ce9-8263-45d0-aa98-deda5cffe3e9
    102. https://pubmed.ncbi.nlm.nih.gov/16762952/

Day 83

    103. https://academic.oup.com/jn/article/133/1/1/4687577#111847234

Day 84

    104. https://www.ncbi.nlm.nih.gov/pmc/articles/PMC5990003/

Day 85

    105. https://liverfoundation.org/for-patients/about-the-liver/health-wellness/nutrition/

Day 86

    106. https://www.todaysdietitian.com/newarchives/060113p40.shtml

Day 87

    107. https://www.nature.com/articles/1602904

Day 88

    108. https://www.ncbi.nlm.nih.gov/pmc/articles/PMC6315720/

Day 89

    109. https://www.ncbi.nlm.nih.gov/pmc/articles/PMC6315720/

Day 90

    110. https://www.ncbi.nlm.nih.gov/pmc/articles/PMC6315720/

Month 4 – Get Outside

Day 91

111. https://www.ncbi.nlm.nih.gov/pmc/articles/PMC2290997/

Day 92

112. https://www.ncbi.nlm.nih.gov/pmc/articles/PMC2290997/

Day 93

113. https://www.ncbi.nlm.nih.gov/pmc/articles/PMC2290997/

Day 94

114. https://www.ncbi.nlm.nih.gov/pmc/articles/PMC2290997/

Day 95

115. https://www.ncbi.nlm.nih.gov/pmc/articles/PMC2290997/

Day 96

116. https://www.ncbi.nlm.nih.gov/pmc/articles/PMC2290997/

Day 97

117. https://www.ncbi.nlm.nih.gov/pmc/articles/PMC2290997/

Day 98

118. https://www.ncbi.nlm.nih.gov/pmc/articles/PMC2290997/

Day 99

119. https://www.ncbi.nlm.nih.gov/pmc/articles/PMC2290997/
120. https://www.ncbi.nlm.nih.gov/pmc/articles/PMC1472821/

Day 100

121. https://www.ncbi.nlm.nih.gov/pmc/articles/PMC2290997/
122. https://www.ncbi.nlm.nih.gov/pmc/articles/PMC6650370/

Day 101

123. https://www.ncbi.nlm.nih.gov/pmc/articles/PMC2290997/

Day 102

124. https://www.ncbi.nlm.nih.gov/pmc/articles/PMC2290997/

Day 103

125. https://www.ncbi.nlm.nih.gov/pmc/articles/PMC2290997/
126. https://pubmed.ncbi.nlm.nih.gov/18698173

Day 104

127. https://www.ncbi.nlm.nih.gov/pmc/articles/PMC2290997/

Day 105

128. https://www.ncbi.nlm.nih.gov/pmc/articles/PMC2290997/

Day 106

129. https://www.ncbi.nlm.nih.gov/pmc/articles/PMC6628736/
130. https://pubmed.ncbi.nlm.nih.gov/28667465/

Day 107

131. https://www.ncbi.nlm.nih.gov/pmc/articles/PMC2290997/

Day 108

132. https://selecthealth.org/blog/2020/07/7-health-benefits-of-sunlight
133. https://www.ncbi.nlm.nih.gov/pmc/articles/PMC6213953/

Day 109

134. https://journals.plos.org/plosone/article?id=10.1371/journal.pone.0092251#s3

Day 110

135. https://www.consumerreports.org/health-wellness/sun-exposure-health-benefits/

Day 111

136. https://www.healthline.com/health/depression/benefits-sunlight#benefits

Day 112

137. https://www.healthline.com/health/depression/benefits-sunlight#benefits

Day 113

138. https://www.healthline.com/health/depression/benefits-sunlight#benefits
139. https://pubmed.ncbi.nlm.nih.gov/27633666/

Day 114

140. https://www.healthline.com/health/depression/benefits-sunlight#benefits
141. https://www.ncbi.nlm.nih.gov/pmc/articles/PMC4999291/

Day 115

142. https://www.theactivetimes.com/healthy-living/15-health-benefits-sunshine/slide-16

Day 116

143. https://yogainternational.com/article/view/5-benefits-of-sunshine

Day 117

144. https://yogainternational.com/article/view/5-benefits-of-sunshine
145. https://www.canr.msu.edu/news/the_benefit_of_daylight_for_our_eyesight

Day 118

146. https://pubmed.ncbi.nlm.nih.gov/27366029

Day 119

147. https://www.ncbi.nlm.nih.gov/pmc/articles/PMC6920963/

Day 120

148. https://www.ncbi.nlm.nih.gov/pmc/articles/PMC7505258/

Month 5 – Grounding

Introduction

149. https://www.ncbi.nlm.nih.gov/pmc/articles/PMC3265077/

Day 121

150. https://www.ncbi.nlm.nih.gov/pmc/articles/PMC3265077/

Day 122

151. https://www.ncbi.nlm.nih.gov/pmc/articles/PMC3265077/

Day 123

152. https://pubmed.ncbi.nlm.nih.gov/30448083/

Day 124

153. https://pubmed.ncbi.nlm.nih.gov/30448083/
154. https://pubmed.ncbi.nlm.nih.gov/25748085/

Day 125

155. https://pubmed.ncbi.nlm.nih.gov/30982019/

Day 126

156. https://chopra.com/articles/grounding-the-human-body-the-healing-benefits-of-earthing

Day 127

157. https://chopra.com/articles/grounding-the-human-body-the-healing-benefits-of-earthing

Day 128

158. https://www.sakara.com/blogs/mag/the-beautiful-benefits-of-grounding
159. https://www.sciencedirect.com/science/article/pii/S1550830719305476

Day 129

160. https://www.sakara.com/blogs/mag/the-beautiful-benefits-of-grounding
161. https://www.ncbi.nlm.nih.gov/pmc/articles/PMC4684131/

Day 130

162. https://www.ncbi.nlm.nih.gov/pmc/articles/PMC4378297/

Day 131

163. https://www.sakara.com/blogs/mag/the-beautiful-benefits-of-grounding

Day 132

164. https://pubmed.ncbi.nlm.nih.gov/25060800/

Day 133

165. https://www.ncbi.nlm.nih.gov/pmc/articles/PMC4590684/

Day 134

166. https://www.sciencedirect.com/science/article/pii/S1550830719305476

Day 135

167. https://www.ncbi.nlm.nih.gov/pmc/articles/PMC3265077/

Day 136

168. https://www.ncbi.nlm.nih.gov/pmc/articles/PMC3151462

Day 137

169. https://www.sciencedirect.com/science/article/pii/S1550830719305476

Day 138

170. https://www.sciencedirect.com/science/article/pii/S1550830719305476

Day 139

171. https://www.netdoctor.co.uk/healthy-living/a33616520/grounding/

Day 140

172. https://www.netdoctor.co.uk/healthy-living/a33616520/grounding/

Day 141

173. https://www.netdoctor.co.uk/healthy-living/a33616520/grounding/

Day 142

174. https://scottjeffrey.com/how-to-ground-yourself/

Day 143

175. https://www.ncbi.nlm.nih.gov/pmc/articles/PMC3779312/

Day 144

176. https://www.huffpost.com/entry/the-healing-benefits-of-grounding-the-human-body_b_592c585be4b07d848fdc058a

Day 145

177. https://www.huffpost.com/entry/the-healing-benefits-of-grounding-the-human-body_b_592c585be4b07d848fdc058a

Day 146

178. https://pubmed.ncbi.nlm.nih.gov/21469913/

Day 147

179. https://www.ncbi.nlm.nih.gov/pmc/articles/PMC4378297/

Day 148

180. https://www.ncbi.nlm.nih.gov/pmc/articles/PMC4378297/

Day 149

181. https://earthinginstitute.net/eyes-vision/

Day 150

182. https://www.ncbi.nlm.nih.gov/pmc/articles/PMC3265077

Month 6 – Park on the Farthest Side of the Parking Lot

Introduction

183. https://www.health.harvard.edu/staying-healthy/walking-your-steps-to-health

Day 151

184. https://www.arthritis.org/health-wellness/healthy-living/physical-activity/walking/12-benefits-of-walking

Day 152

185. https://www.arthritis.org/health-wellness/healthy-living/physical-activity/walking/12-benefits-of-walking

Day 153

186. https://www.arthritis.org/health-wellness/healthy-living/physical-activity/walking/12-benefits-of-walking
187. https://www.healthline.com/health/benefits-of-walking#increased-life-span

Day 154

188. https://www.arthritis.org/health-wellness/healthy-living/physical-activity/walking/12-benefits-of-walking
189. https://www.healthline.com/health/benefits-of-walking#mood-enhancer

Day 155

190. https://www.arthritis.org/health-wellness/healthy-living/physical-activity/walking/12-benefits-of-walking

Day 156

191. https://www.arthritis.org/health-wellness/healthy-living/physical-activity/walking/12-benefits-of-walking
192. https://www.healthline.com/health/benefits-of-walking#muscle-tone

Day 157

193. https://www.arthritis.org/health-wellness/healthy-living/physical-activity/walking/12-benefits-of-walking
194. https://www.sciencedirect.com/science/article/abs/pii/S2352721819301056?via%3Dihub

Day 158

195. https://www.arthritis.org/health-wellness/healthy-living/physical-activity/walking/12-benefits-of-walking
196. https://www.healthline.com/health/benefits-of-walking#joint-pain

Day 159

197. https://www.arthritis.org/health-wellness/healthy-living/physical-activity/walking/12-benefits-of-walking
198. https://www.healthline.com/health/benefits-of-walking#energy-boost

Day 160

199. https://www.arthritis.org/health-wellness/healthy-living/physical-activity/walking/12-benefits-of-walking

Day 161

200. https://www.arthritis.org/health-wellness/healthy-living/physical-activity/walking/12-benefits-of-walking

Day 162

201. https://www.healthline.com/health/benefits-of-walking#immunity

Day 163

202. https://www.healthline.com/health/benefits-of-walking#immunity

Day 164

203. https://psycnet.apa.org/record/2014-14435-001

Day 165

204. https://www.prevention.com/fitness/a20485587/benefits-from-walking-every-day/

Day 166

205. https://www.prevention.com/fitness/a20485587/benefits-from-walking-every-day/

Day 167

206. https://www.health.harvard.edu/staying-healthy/5-surprising-benefits-of-walking

Day 168

207. https://www.health.harvard.edu/staying-healthy/5-surprising-benefits-of-walking

Day 169

208. https://www.health.harvard.edu/staying-healthy/5-surprising-benefits-of-walking

Day 170

209. https://www.cancer.gov/about-cancer/causes-prevention/risk/obesity/physical-activity-fact-sheet

Day 171

210. https://www.wisemanfamilypractice.com/health-benefits-sweating/

Day 172

211. https://www.dummies.com/health/exercise/cardio/how-walking-can-increase-flexibility

Day 173

212. https://jamanetwork.com/journals/jama/fullarticle/195504

Day 174

213. https://www.aaaai.org/conditions-and-treatments/library/asthma-library/exercise-and-asthma

Day 175

214. https://www.thehealthy.com/exercise/walking/walking-benefits-15-minutes/

Day 176

215. https://www.thehealthy.com/exercise/walking/walking-benefits-15-minutes/

Day 177

216. https://www.thehealthy.com/exercise/walking/walking-benefits-15-minutes/

Day 178

217. https://www.realbuzz.com/articles-interests/walking/article/10-big-health-benefits-of-walking/

Day 179

218. https://www.healthifyme.com/blog/13-health-benefits-of-walking/

Day 180

219. https://www.healthifyme.com/blog/13-health-benefits-of-walking/

Month 7 – Keep Magnesium Spray in the Shower

Introduction

220. https://www.ncbi.nlm.nih.gov/pmc/articles/PMC1855626/

Day 181

221. https://betteryou.com/magnesium
222. https://www.healthline.com/health/magnesium-oil-benefits#side-effects-and-risks

Day 182

223. https://www.ncbi.nlm.nih.gov/books/NBK507250/

Day 183

224. https://www.nps.org.au/news/magnesium-a-treatment-for-leg-cramps
225. https://www.clinicaltrials.gov/ct2/show/study/NCT00963638

Day 184

226. https://ods.od.nih.gov/factsheets/Magnesium-HealthProfessional/

Day 185

227. https://www.ncbi.nlm.nih.gov/pmc/articles/PMC6024559/

Day 186

228. https://www.ncbi.nlm.nih.gov/pmc/articles/PMC4062555/

Day 187

229. https://www.healthline.com/health/arrhythmia/alternative-treatments

Day 188

230. https://www.ncbi.nlm.nih.gov/pmc/articles/PMC6024559/

Day 189

231. https://www.ncbi.nlm.nih.gov/pmc/articles/PMC6024559/
232. https://pubmed.ncbi.nlm.nih.gov/27807012/

Day 190

233. https://www.ncbi.nlm.nih.gov/pmc/articles/PMC2464251/

Day 191

234. https://www.ncbi.nlm.nih.gov/pmc/articles/PMC5794996/
235. https://share.upmc.com/2018/09/what-is-vascular-calcification/

Day 192

236. https://share.upmc.com/2018/09/what-is-vascular-calcification/

Day 193

237. https://www.webmd.com/alzheimers/news/20170920/high-low-magnesium-levels-tied-to-dementia-risk#1

Day 194

238. https://www.ackdjournal.org/article/S1548-5595(17)30202-1/pdf#:~:text=Magnesium%20deficiency%20is%20known%20to,to%20end%2Dstage%20kidney%20disease

Day 195

239. https://www.ncbi.nlm.nih.gov/books/NBK507266/

Day 196

240. https://www.ncbi.nlm.nih.gov/pmc/articles/PMC5579607/
241. https://www.ncbi.nlm.nih.gov/pmc/articles/PMC5590399/

Day 197

242. https://www.ncbi.nlm.nih.gov/pmc/articles/PMC5579607/

Day 198

243. https://www.medicalnewstoday.com/articles/323755
244. https://www.ncbi.nlm.nih.gov/pmc/articles/PMC3269605/

Day 199

245. https://www.ncbi.nlm.nih.gov/pmc/articles/PMC3775240/#B11-nutrients-05-03022
246. https://pubmed.ncbi.nlm.nih.gov/19828898/

Day 200

247. https://www.healthline.com/health/gerd/magnesium-acid-reflux

Day 201

248. https://www.fgb.com.au/content/magnesium-deficiency

Day 202

249. https://www.fgb.com.au/content/magnesium-deficiency

Day 203

250. https://www.ncbi.nlm.nih.gov/pmc/articles/PMC3208934/

Day 204

251. https://www.fgb.com.au/content/magnesium-deficiency

Day 205

252. https://www.ncbi.nlm.nih.gov/pmc/articles/PMC4897098/

Day 206

253. https://www.ncbi.nlm.nih.gov/pmc/articles/PMC6153988/
254. https://www.growinggrins.com/blog/2018/12/17/5-important-vitamins-and-minerals-for-healthy-teeth#:~:text=Magnesium%20is%20a%20fantastic%20mineral,strong%20teeth%20and%20tooth%20enamel

Day 207

255. https://www.medicalnewstoday.com/articles/322191
256. https://www.ncbi.nlm.nih.gov/books/NBK519036/

Day 208

257. https://www.ncbi.nlm.nih.gov/pmc/articles/PMC5417264/

Day 209

258. https://ods.od.nih.gov/factsheets/Magnesium-HealthProfessional/

Day 210

259. https://www.ncbi.nlm.nih.gov/pmc/articles/PMC4283390/

Month 8 – Ashwagandha

Day 211

260. https://pubmed.ncbi.nlm.nih.gov/19633611/
261. https://en.wikipedia.org/wiki/Withaferin_A#Anti-tumor
262. https://www.ncbi.nlm.nih.gov/pmc/articles/PMC3252722/

Day 212

263. https://en.wikipedia.org/wiki/Withaferin_A#Anti-inflammatory

Day 213

264. https://en.wikipedia.org/wiki/Withaferin_A#Clinical_relevance

Day 214

265. https://en.wikipedia.org/wiki/Withaferin_A#Clinical_relevance

Day 215

266. https://www.ncbi.nlm.nih.gov/pmc/articles/PMC5871210/
267. https://pubmed.ncbi.nlm.nih.gov/21407960/
268. https://www.ncbi.nlm.nih.gov/pmc/articles/PMC3573577/

Day 216

269. https://examine.com/supplements/ashwagandha/

Day 217

270. https://www.ncbi.nlm.nih.gov/pmc/articles/PMC5871210/

Day 218

271. https://pubmed.ncbi.nlm.nih.gov/26527154/

Day 219

272. https://www.ncbi.nlm.nih.gov/pmc/articles/PMC4658772/

Day 220

273. https://pubmed.ncbi.nlm.nih.gov/25796090/

Day 221

274. https://pubmed.ncbi.nlm.nih.gov/19789214/
275. https://pubmed.ncbi.nlm.nih.gov/23796876/
276. https://pubmed.ncbi.nlm.nih.gov/19501822/

Day 222

277. https://www.ncbi.nlm.nih.gov/pmc/articles/PMC6438434/

Day 223

278. https://pubmed.ncbi.nlm.nih.gov/16713218/

Day 224

279. https://pubmed.ncbi.nlm.nih.gov/22700086/
280. https://pubmed.ncbi.nlm.nih.gov/28471731/
281. https://pubmed.ncbi.nlm.nih.gov/24497737/

Day 225

282. https://pubmed.ncbi.nlm.nih.gov/27037574/

Day 226

283. https://www.ncbi.nlm.nih.gov/pmc/articles/PMC3252722/

Day 227

284. https://www.ncbi.nlm.nih.gov/pmc/articles/PMC3252722/
285. https://pubmed.ncbi.nlm.nih.gov/16387694/

Day 228

286. https://www.ncbi.nlm.nih.gov/pmc/articles/PMC3252722/

Day 229

287. https://www.ncbi.nlm.nih.gov/pmc/articles/PMC3252722/
288. https://www.healthline.com/nutrition/12-proven-ashwagandha-benefits#7

Day 230

289. https://www.ncbi.nlm.nih.gov/pmc/articles/PMC3252722/
290. https://www.nutraingredients.com/Article/2016/11/23/Ashwagandha-root-extracts-shows-anti-aging-effect-Cell-study#

Day 231

291. https://www.ncbi.nlm.nih.gov/pmc/articles/PMC3252722/
292. https://pubmed.ncbi.nlm.nih.gov/25857501/

Day 232

293. https://www.ncbi.nlm.nih.gov/pmc/articles/PMC3252722/

Day 233

294. https://pubmed.ncbi.nlm.nih.gov/24330893/

Day 234

295. https://pubmed.ncbi.nlm.nih.gov/23142798/

Day 235

296. https://www.webmd.com/vitamins/ai/ingredientmono-953/ashwagandha
297. https://pubmed.ncbi.nlm.nih.gov/27515872/

Day 236

298. https://examine.com/supplements/ashwagandha/
299. https://pubmed.ncbi.nlm.nih.gov/21170205/

Day 237

300. https://examine.com/supplements/ashwagandha/

Day 238

301. https://examine.com/supplements/ashwagandha/

Day 239

302. https://examine.com/supplements/ashwagandha/

Day 240

303. https://examine.com/supplements/ashwagandha/
304. https://www.ncbi.nlm.nih.gov/pmc/articles/PMC3573577/

Month 9 – Wear Blue Blockers (Light Timing)

Day 241

305. https://pubmed.ncbi.nlm.nih.gov/16842544/

Day 242

306. https://www.ncbi.nlm.nih.gov/pmc/articles/PMC6211454/

Day 243

307. https://www.ncbi.nlm.nih.gov/pmc/articles/PMC6211454/
308. https://pubmed.ncbi.nlm.nih.gov/20030543/

Day 244

309. https://pubmed.ncbi.nlm.nih.gov/21300732/

Day 245

310. https://pubmed.ncbi.nlm.nih.gov/19910503/

Day 246

311. https://pubmed.ncbi.nlm.nih.gov/23814343/

Day 247

312. https://pubmed.ncbi.nlm.nih.gov/23814343/

Day 248

313. https://pubmed.ncbi.nlm.nih.gov/23814343/

Day 249

314. https://www.ncbi.nlm.nih.gov/pmc/articles/PMC2398753/

Day 250

315. https://pubmed.ncbi.nlm.nih.gov/23946702/

Day 251

316. https://www.healthline.com/health/sleep-deprivation/effects-on-body
317. https://pubmed.ncbi.nlm.nih.gov/4345657/

Day 252

318. https://www.healthline.com/health/sleep-deprivation/effects-on-body

Day 253

319. https://www.healthline.com/health/sleep-deprivation/effects-on-body

Day 254

320. https://www.healthline.com/health/sleep-deprivation/effects-on-body

Day 255

321. https://www.healthline.com/health/sleep-deprivation/effects-on-body

Day 256

322. https://www.healthline.com/health/sleep-deprivation/effects-on-body

Day 257

323. https://www.webmd.com/sleep-disorders/features/10-results-sleep-loss
324. https://pubmed.ncbi.nlm.nih.gov/25266053/

Day 258

325. https://www.webmd.com/sleep-disorders/features/10-results-sleep-loss

Day 259

326. https://www.ncbi.nlm.nih.gov/pmc/articles/PMC4970273/

Day 260

327. https://www.medicalnewstoday.com/articles/307334#what-people-need

Day 261

328. https://www.medicalnewstoday.com/articles/307334#effects-on-the-body

Day 262

329. https://www.ncbi.nlm.nih.gov/pmc/articles/PMC5749041/

Day 263

330. https://www.medicalnewstoday.com/articles/307334#causes

Day 264

331. https://www.ncbi.nlm.nih.gov/pmc/articles/PMC5449130/

Day 265

332. https://www.hopkinsmedicine.org/health/wellness-and-prevention/the-effects-of-sleep-deprivation

Day 266

333. https://www.orthodonticslimited.com/your-health/lack-sleep-dangerous-dental-health/#:~:text=Studies%20have%20shown%20that%20the,holds%20your%20teeth%20in%20place

Day 267

334. https://www.hopkinsmedicine.org/health/wellness-and-prevention/the-effects-of-sleep-deprivation

Day 268

335. https://www.hopkinsmedicine.org/health/wellness-and-prevention/the-effects-of-sleep-deprivation

Day 269

336. https://www.ncbi.nlm.nih.gov/books/NBK19961/

Day 270

337. https://www.betterhealth.vic.gov.au/health/conditionsandtreatments/sleep-deprivation

Month 10 – Breathing

Day 271

338. https://lunginstitute.com/blog/oxygen-levels-digestive-system/

Day 272

339. https://www.kent-teach.com/Blog/post/2017/04/25/6-benefits-of-getting-fresh-air.aspx

Day 273

340. https://www.ncbi.nlm.nih.gov/books/NBK232882/

Day 274

341. https://www.kent-teach.com/Blog/post/2017/04/25/6-benefits-of-getting-fresh-air.aspx

Day 275

342. https://www.kent-teach.com/Blog/post/2017/04/25/6-benefits-of-getting-fresh-air.aspx

Day 276

343. https://www.kent-teach.com/Blog/post/2017/04/25/6-benefits-of-getting-fresh-air.aspx

Day 277

344. https://valeowc.com/the-benefits-of-oxygen/

Day 278

345. https://thorax.bmj.com/content/59/8/668

Day 279

346. https://www.terrapinadventures.com/blog/exercise-fresh-air-health/
347. https://www.bbc.com/future/article/20151207-the-air-that-makes-you-fat

Day 280

348. https://physiofalmouthplus.co.uk/health-benefits-fresh-air/

281

349. https://www.webmd.com/lung/lung-diseases-overview
350. https://www.independent.co.uk/news/uk/fresh-air-best-cure-asthma-1532321.html

Day 282

351. https://valeowc.com/the-benefits-of-oxygen/

Day 283

352. https://valeowc.com/the-benefits-of-oxygen/

Day 284

353. https://valeowc.com/the-benefits-of-oxygen/

Day 285

354. https://pubmed.ncbi.nlm.nih.gov/1237867/

Day 286

355. https://valeowc.com/the-benefits-of-oxygen/

Day 287

356. https://valeowc.com/the-benefits-of-oxygen/

Day 288

357. https://valeowc.com/the-benefits-of-oxygen/

Day 289

358. https://valeowc.com/the-benefits-of-oxygen/

Day 290

359. https://pubmed.ncbi.nlm.nih.gov/15086128/

Day 291

360. https://www.ncbi.nlm.nih.gov/pmc/articles/PMC4818249/

Day 292

361. https://www.oxygenworldwide.com/news/articles-and-information/662-general-benefits-of-oxygen.html

Day 293

362. https://www.oxygenworldwide.com/news/articles-and-information/662-general-benefits-of-oxygen.html

Day 294

363. https://www.ncbi.nlm.nih.gov/pmc/articles/PMC3930928/

Day 295

364. https://www.abc.net.au/health/talkinghealth/factbuster/stories/2012/07/24/3552405.htm

Day 296

365. https://pubmed.ncbi.nlm.nih.gov/10757682/

Day 297

366. https://www.lung.org/blog/lung-cancer-and-pollution

Day 298

367. https://my.clevelandclinic.org/health/diseases/17727-hypoxemia

Day 299

368. https://www.oxygenworldwide.com/news/articles-and-information/662-general-benefits-of-oxygen.html

Day 300

369. https://www.webmd.com/lung/lung-home-oxygen-therapy

Month 11 – Meditate

Day 301

    370. https://www.mayoclinic.org/tests-procedures/meditation/in-depth/meditation/art-20045858

Day 302

    371. https://www.mayoclinic.org/tests-procedures/meditation/in-depth/meditation/art-20045858

Day 303

    372. https://www.mayoclinic.org/tests-procedures/meditation/in-depth/meditation/art-20045858

Day 304

    373. https://www.mayoclinic.org/tests-procedures/meditation/in-depth/meditation/art-20045858

Day 305

    374. https://www.mayoclinic.org/tests-procedures/meditation/in-depth/meditation/art-20045858

Day 306

    375. https://www.mayoclinic.org/tests-procedures/meditation/in-depth/meditation/art-20045858
    376. https://www.ncbi.nlm.nih.gov/pmc/articles/PMC3887545/

Day 307

    377. https://www.mayoclinic.org/tests-procedures/meditation/in-depth/meditation/art-20045858

Day 308

    378. https://www.mayoclinic.org/tests-procedures/meditation/in-depth/meditation/art-20045858

Day 309

    379. https://www.mayoclinic.org/tests-procedures/meditation/in-depth/meditation/art-20045858

Day 310

    380. https://www.mayoclinic.org/tests-procedures/meditation/in-depth/meditation/art-20045858

Day 311

    381. https://www.mayoclinic.org/tests-procedures/meditation/in-depth/meditation/art-20045858

Day 312

    382. https://www.mayoclinic.org/tests-procedures/meditation/in-depth/meditation/art-20045858

Day 313

    383. https://www.mayoclinic.org/tests-procedures/meditation/in-depth/meditation/art-20045858

Day 314

    384. https://www.mayoclinic.org/tests-procedures/meditation/in-depth/meditation/art-20045858

Day 315

    385. https://www.mayoclinic.org/tests-procedures/meditation/in-depth/meditation/art-20045858

Day 316

    386. https://www.mayoclinic.org/tests-procedures/meditation/in-depth/meditation/art-20045858

Day 317

    387. https://www.mayoclinic.org/tests-procedures/meditation/in-depth/meditation/art-20045858

Day 318

    388. https://www.mayoclinic.org/tests-procedures/meditation/in-depth/meditation/art-20045858

Day 319

    389. https://www.mayoclinic.org/tests-procedures/meditation/in-depth/meditation/art-20045858

Day 320

    390. https://www.mayoclinic.org/tests-procedures/meditation/in-depth/meditation/art-20045858

Day 321

391. https://www.mayoclinic.org/tests-procedures/meditation/in-depth/meditation/art-20045858
392. https://www.ncbi.nlm.nih.gov/pmc/articles/PMC6088366/

Day 322

393. https://pubmed.ncbi.nlm.nih.gov/29619620/

Day 323

394. https://pubmed.ncbi.nlm.nih.gov/27537781/

Day 324

395. https://pubmed.ncbi.nlm.nih.gov/30153464/

Day 325

396. https://pubmed.ncbi.nlm.nih.gov/26445019/

Day 326

397. https://pubmed.ncbi.nlm.nih.gov/24571182/

Day 327

398. https://pubmed.ncbi.nlm.nih.gov/24093954/

Day 328

399. https://pubmed.ncbi.nlm.nih.gov/24979314/

Day 329

400. https://www.ncbi.nlm.nih.gov/pmc/articles/PMC6081743/

Day 330

401. https://www.healthline.com/nutrition/12-benefits-of-meditation#8.-May-help-fight-addictions

Month 12 – Practice a Daily Affirmation

Day 331

    402. https://theblissfulmind.com/positive-affirmations-list

Day 332

    403. https://theblissfulmind.com/positive-affirmations-list

Day 333

    404. https://theblissfulmind.com/positive-affirmations-list

Day 334

    405. https://theblissfulmind.com/positive-affirmations-list

Day 335

    406. https://theblissfulmind.com/positive-affirmations-list

Day 336

    407. https://theblissfulmind.com/positive-affirmations-list

Day 337

    408. https://theblissfulmind.com/positive-affirmations-list

Day 338

    409. https://theblissfulmind.com/positive-affirmations-list

Day 339

    410. https://theblissfulmind.com/positive-affirmations-list

Day 340

    411. https://theblissfulmind.com/positive-affirmations-list

Day 341

    412. https://theblissfulmind.com/positive-affirmations-list

Day 342

    413. https://theblissfulmind.com/positive-affirmations-list

Day 343

    414. https://theblissfulmind.com/positive-affirmations-list

Day 344

415. https://theblissfulmind.com/positive-affirmations-list

Day 345

416. https://theblissfulmind.com/positive-affirmations-list

Day 346

417. https://theblissfulmind.com/positive-affirmations-list

Day 347

418. https://theblissfulmind.com/positive-affirmations-list

Day 348

419. https://theblissfulmind.com/positive-affirmations-list

Day 349

420. https://theblissfulmind.com/positive-affirmations-list

Day 350

421. https://theblissfulmind.com/positive-affirmations-list

Day 351

422. https://theblissfulmind.com/positive-affirmations-list

Day 352

423. https://theblissfulmind.com/positive-affirmations-list

Day 353

424. https://theblissfulmind.com/positive-affirmations-list

Day 354

425. https://theblissfulmind.com/positive-affirmations-list

Day 355

426. https://theblissfulmind.com/positive-affirmations-list

Day 356

427. https://www.huffpost.com/entry/affirmations_b_3527028

Day 357

428. https://www.huffpost.com/entry/affirmations_b_3527028

Day 358

429. https://www.huffpost.com/entry/affirmations_b_3527028

Day 359

430. https://www.huffpost.com/entry/affirmations_b_3527028

Day 360

431. https://www.huffpost.com/entry/affirmations_b_3527028

We Want to Hear from You!

Reviews are an important part of how others find our books, and they help us create content you love. If you enjoyed this book, please visit the associated Amazon product listing and leave us a review. We will use your feedback to help create more content catered toward you, our loyal readers.

Thank you!!

whistlekick Training Programs

Looking to increase your speed? How about your fighting endurance? Visit whistlekick.com to see how we are revolutionizing the way you train to improve not only your martial arts skills, but also your overall health.

Just released – the FREE whistlekick Flexibility Program!

Yes, I said FREE! This program is designed by and for martial artists with features you won't find in any other program, at any price. The Flexibility Program is rooted in the latest science, immensely effective, and different from what most of us were taught.

Check out the collection of whistlekick Programs in the whistlekick Store today!

We Truly Appreciate You!

Thank you for supporting whistlekick Books. We invite you to visit us at whistlekick.com/family, a webpage designed especially for our whistlekick family members, like you. While there, you will find links to check out our other books, our store, social media, how to leave us reviews, info on our other projects, and much more.

We are always open to your thoughts, questions, and suggestions. You may contact us anytime at info@whistlekick.com.

Thank you!

Made in the USA
Coppell, TX
26 August 2022

82080880R00246